DEDICATION

We dedicate this volume to our diabetic patients and to all those who work to prevent and control type 2 diabetes

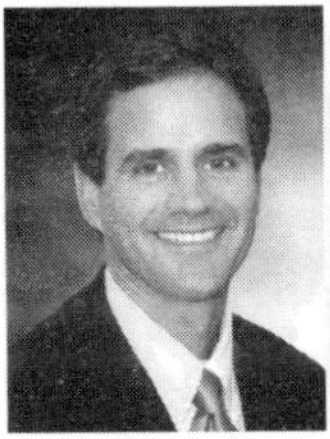

James H. O'Keefe, Jr, MD

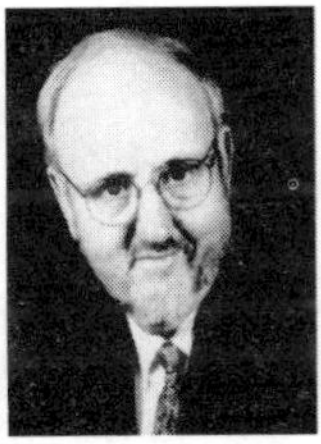

David S. H. Bell, MB

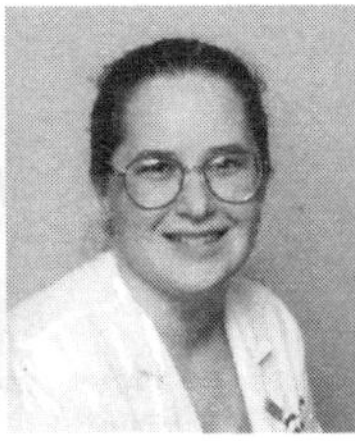

Kathleen L. Wyne, MD, PhD

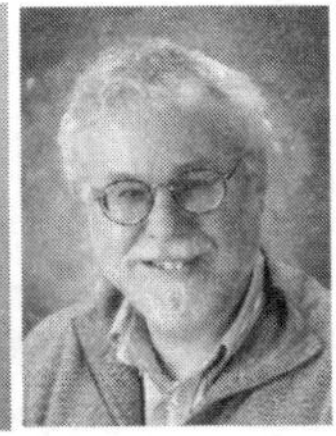

Steven M. Haffner, MD

TABLES AND FIGURES

DIABETES ESSENTIALS

Third Edition

James H. O'Keefe, Jr., MD
Director, Preventive Cardiology
Mid-America Heart Institute
Clinical Professor of Medicine
University of Missouri School of Medicine
Kansas City, Missouri

David S. H. Bell, MB
Clinical Professor of Medicine
University of Alabama at Birmingham School of Medicine
Birmingham, Alabama

Kathleen L. Wyne, MD, PhD
Assistant Professor of Medicine
Division of Endocrinology and Metabolism
University of Texas Southwestern Medical Center
Dallas, Texas

Steven M. Haffner, MD
Professor of Medicine
University of Texas Health Sciences Center at San Antonio
San Antonio, Texas

PHYSICIANS' PRESS

Innovative Medical Publishing

ABOUT THE AUTHORS

James H. O'Keefe, Jr., M.D., is Director of Preventive Cardiology at the Mid America Heart Institute and Professor of Medicine at the University of Missouri in Kansas City. His postgraduate training included a cardiology fellowship at Mayo Clinic in Rochester, Minnesota. He has written 150 articles and 6 books on cardiovascular medicine, and he lectures extensively on the role of therapeutic lifestyle changes and drug therapy in cardiovascular risk reduction. He is actively involved in patient care.

David S. H. Bell, MB, is a Clinical Professor of Medicine at the University of Alabama at Birmingham, School of Medicine, and is a leading authority on the prevention and treatment of type 2 diabetes. During his distinguished career, he has contributed more than 240 articles to the medical literature. He is an active researcher and has served as Director of the Endocrine Clinical Research Program at the University of Alabama Birmingham. Dr. Bell speaks nationally and internationally on the treatment of type 2 diabetes and its complications, and he is currently or has been a member of the editorial boards of *Endocrine Practice*, *Treatments in Endocrinology*, *Diabetes*, and *Obesity and Metabolism*. He is a recipient of the Distinguished Clinician Award from the American College of Endocrinology for outstanding contribution as a master educator and clinician and the Seale Harris Award from the Southern Medical Association for superior contributions to the art and science of diabetes and endocrinology.

Kathleen L. Wyne, MD, PhD, is an Assistant Professor in the Division of Endocrinology and Metabolism at the University of Texas Southwestern Medical Center, Dallas, Texas. She is actively involved in basic science and clinical research, and her main research interests include the role of lipid metabolism in the etiology of diabetes and genetic causes of beta cell defects. In 1999 she received a Career Development Award from the Juvenile Diabetes Research Foundation International, and in 2000 she received a research grant from the same organization. Dr. Wyne has contributed many articles to the medical literature and lectures extensively on lipid metabolism and diabetes treatment. She is actively involved in patient care.

Steven M. Haffner, MD, is Professor of Medicine at the University of Texas Health Sciences Center at San Antonio and is one of the world's leading authorities on diabetes. He has contributed more than 330 articles to the medical literature and speaks nationally and internationally on insulin resistance, the metabolic syndrome, and treatment of type 2 diabetes. He is currently a member of the editorial boards of *Diabetes, Circulation*, and the *Journal of Clinical Endocrinology and Metabolism.* Dr. Haffner served on the American Diabetes Association's Professional Practices Committee from 2000-2002 and has been a consultant for the National Cholesterol Education Program sections on the metabolic syndrome and diabetes. He is a recipient of the Kelly West Award from the American Diabetes Association for his outstanding contribution to diabetes epidemiology. He is an active researcher and has been elected to the American Society of Clinical Investigators. His main research interest is in insulin resistance and type 2 diabetes.

 Additional copies of *Diabetes Essentials* can be obtained at medical bookstores or by contacting Physicians' Press, 620 Cherry Street, Royal Oak, Michigan, 48073; telephone: (248) 616-3023; fax: (248) 616-3003; visit www.physicianspress.com.

Printed in the United States of America ISBN: 978-1-890114-67-1

TABLE OF CONTENTS

CONTRIBUTORS

David S. H. Bell, MB
Clinical Professor of Medicine
University of Alabama Birmingham
Birmingham, Alabama

George L. Bakris, MD†
Professor of Preventive Medicine
Director, Hypertension/Clinical Research Center
Rush University Medical Center
Chicago, Illinois

Christie M. Ballantyne, MD*
Clinical Director, Section of Atherosclerosis
Professor of Medicine
Baylor College of Medicine
Houston, Texas

Mark S. Freed, MD
Cardiologist
President and Editor-in-Chief
Physicians' Press
Royal Oak, Michigan

Steven M. Haffner, MD
Professor of Medicine
University of Texas Health Sciences Center
San Antonio, Texas

Janet Haskin, PharmD
Clinical Coordinator
Del Sol Medical Center
El Paso, Texas
Diabetes Drug Summaries

Antonio M. Gotto, Jr, MD, DPhil*
The Stephen and Suzanne Weiss Dean
Professor of Medicine
Provost for Medical Affairs
The Weill Medical College of Cornell University
New York, New York

James H. O'Keefe, Jr, MD
Director, Preventive Cardiology
Mid America Heart Institute
Clinical Professor of Medicine
University of Missouri School of Medicine
Kansas City, Missouri

David M. Safley, MD
Cardiologist
Mid America Heart Institute
Kansas City, Missouri
Clinical Trials

Kathleen L. Wyne, MD, PhD
Assistant Professor
Division of Endocrinology and Metabolism
University of Texas Southwestern Medical Center
Dallas, Texas

---

* Portions of Chapter 7, "Control of Dyslipidemia in Type 2 Diabetes," and Chapter 9, "Other Measures to Reduce Atherothrombosis," from *Dyslipidemia Essentials*, by Ballantyne CM, O'Keefe JH, Jr, Gotto AM, Jr, Physicians' Press, 2007, Royal Oak, Michigan

† Portions of Chapter 8, "Control of Hypertension in Type 2 Diabetes," from *Handbook of Diabetic Hypertension*, by Bell DSH, O'Keefe JH, Jr, Bakris GL, Physicians' Press, 2006, Royal Oak, Michigan

ACKNOWLEDGMENTS

To accomplish the task of presenting the data compiled in this reference, a small, dedicated team of professionals was assembled. We wish to acknowledge Monica Crowder Kaufman for her important contribution, Norman Lyle for cover design, Bradley Melnick and Josephine Sydney Greenberg for their assistance, and Mark S. Freed, MD, President and Editor-in-Chief of Physicians' Press, for his vision, commitment, and guidance.

James H. O'Keefe, Jr, MD
Kathleen L. Wyne, MD, PhD
David S.H. Bell, MB
Steven M. Haffner, MD

NOTICE

Diabetes Essentials has been developed as a concise, practical, and authoritative guide tor the treatment of patients with type 2 diabetes mellitus. The clinical recommendations set forth in this book are those of the authors and are offered as general guidelines, not specific instructions for individual patients. Clinical judgment should always guide the physician in the selection, dosing, and duration of drug therapy for individual patients. Not all medications have been accepted by the U.S. Food and Drug Administration for indications cited in this book, and drug recommendations are not necessarily limited to indications in the package insert. The use of any drug should be preceded by careful review of the package insert, which provides indications and dosing approved by the U.S. Food and Drug Administration. The information provided in this book is not exhaustive, and the reader is referred to other medical references and the manufacturer's product literature for further information. Clinical use of the information provided and any consequences that may arise from its use is the responsibility of the prescribing physician. The authors, editors, and publisher do not warrant or guarantee the information herein contained, and do not assume and expressly disclaim any liability for errors or omissions or any consequences that may occur from use of this information.

ABBREVIATIONS

AACE/ACE American Association of Clinical Endocrinologists/American College of Endocrinology
ACE angiotensin converting enzyme
ACS acute coronary syndrome
ADA American Diabetes Association
ADP adenosine diphosphate
AHA American Heart Association
ARB angiotensin receptor blocker
ATP Adult Treatment Panel (National Cholesterol Education Program)
BID twice daily
BMI body mass index
BP blood pressure
BUN blood urea nitrogen
CABG coronary artery bypass grafting
CHD coronary heart disease
CI contraindication
CK creatine kinase
CNS central nervous system
COPD chronic obstructive pulmonary disease
CrCl creatinine clearance
CRP C-reactive protein
DHA docosahexaenoic acid
DKA diabetic ketoacidosis
dL deciliter
DPP-4 dipeptidyl peptidase-4
DVT deep venous thrombosis
ECG electrocardiogram
e.g. for example
EPA eicosapentaenoic acid
FBG fasting blood glucose
FDA Food and Drug Administration
FPG fasting plasma glucose
g gram
GDM gestational diabetes mellitus
GI gastrointestinal
GIP glucose-dependent insulinotropic polypeptide
GLP-1 glucagon-like peptide-1
gm gram
GFR glomerular filtration rate
GP glycoprotein
HbA_{1c} hemoglobin A_{1c}
HDL high-density lipoprotein
Hg hemoglobin
IFG impaired fasting glucose
IGT impaired glucose tolerance
IV intravenous
kg kilogram
L liter
LDL low-density lipoprotein
LFT liver function test
Lp(a) lipoprotein(a)
LV left ventricular; left ventricle
LVH left ventricular hypertrophy
max maximum
cg microgram
mcL microliter
mg milligram
MI myocardial infarction
min minute
mL milliliter
NCEP National Cholesterol Education Program
NRT nicotine replacement therapy
NYHA New York Heart Association
O_2 oxygen
OGTT oral glucose tolerance test
PAI-1 plasminogen activator inhibitor-1
PCI percutaneous coronary intervention
PE pulmonary embolism
PO per os - by mouth; oral
PPAR peroxisome proliferator-activated receptor
q__h every __ hours
q__d every __ days
RCT randomized controlled trial
TG triglyceride
TIA transient ischemic attack
TLC therapeutic lifestyle changes
TID three times daily
TZD thiazolidinedione
US United States

Chapter 1

Diabetes Essentials

Diabetes mellitus is a global public health problem of epidemic proportions, and its incidence is on the rise. In the United States (US) alone, approximately 21 million adults have diabetes and 35% of adults have prediabetes or diabetes (Diabetes Care 2006;29:1263-1268). Worldwide, more than 150 million adults have diabetes, a number the World Health Organization expects to double over the next 20 years.

Diabetes is associated with accelerated atherosclerosis and a prothrombotic state, markedly increasing the risk of myocardial infarction (MI), stroke, peripheral arterial disease, and heart failure. Seventy-five percent of individuals with diabetes die from cardiovascular disease, and diabetic subjects without known coronary artery disease have the same cardiovascular prognosis as nondiabetic subjects with coronary artery disease. Of patients admitted to hospitals in the US, 43% have diabetes. Diabetes is also the leading cause of adult blindness, end-stage renal disease, and nontraumatic leg amputation. Diabetes confers an equivalent cardiovascular risk to aging 15 years (Lancet 2006;368:29-36). Compared to death rates for cardiovascular disease, stroke, and cancer, which have remained stable or have declined since 1980, death rates for diabetes have increased by 30% during the same time period. The annual cost of diabetes in terms of medical care and lost productivity exceeds $130 billion in the United States alone.

Measures aimed at slowing the progression of atherosclerosis, stabilizing rupture-prone plaques, and preventing arterial thrombosis can reduce the risk of cardiac death, MI, stroke, revascularization procedures, and peripheral arterial disease by 50%-80%. The lower the hemoglobin A_{1c}, even within the normal range, the lower the risk of a cardiovascular event and cardiac and all-cause mortality. Despite these benefits, only 7.3% of individuals with diabetes meet national guidelines for control of hemoglobin A_{1c}, cholesterol and blood pressure, and tens of thousands of lives are lost each year from failure to implement established measures. The American Diabetes Association (ADA) has estimated that, in the US alone, if 80% of individuals with type 2 diabetes achieved five recommended ADA treatment goals over

Table 1.1. ADA Treatment Goals for Individuals with Type 2 Diabetes

- Hemoglobin A1c < 7%
- Blood pressure < 130/80 mmHg
- LDL cholesterol < 100 mg/dL
- HDL > 40 mg/dL for men and > 50 mg/dL for women
- Use of aspirin, 81 mg daily

the next 30 years (Table 1.1), there would be 5 million fewer heart attacks, 1.2 million fewer cases of kidney failure, 1.8 million fewer cases of blindness, and 1.8 million fewer premature deaths. In addition, more than $150 billion in medical costs could be saved. *Diabetes Essentials* incorporates the latest guidelines and trials into a practical, concise, authoritative guide to the diagnosis, evaluation, prevention, and management of type 2 diabetes, the most prevalent form of the disease.

Overview of Diabetes Mellitus

A. **Description.** Diabetes mellitus is the most common endocrine disorder in men and women. It is caused by an absolute lack of insulin (type 1) or a relative lack of insulin (type 2) that is insufficient to overcome insulin resistance. Manifestations include hyperglycemia, other metabolic derangements, and long-term damage to blood vessels, eyes, nerves, kidneys, and the heart (Table 1.2). Diabetes is a leading cause of cardiac death, nonfatal MI, heart failure, and stroke; it is also the most common cause of adult blindness, end-stage renal disease, nontraumatic leg amputation, and neuropathy in the United States.

B. **Prevalence.** Approximately 21 million Americans and 150 million individuals worldwide have diabetes, a number projected to double by the year 2025. Over a 10-year period from 1990-2000, the prevalence of diabetes increased by 49%, from 4.9% to 7.3% in the US. The US Centers for Disease Control and Prevention estimates that in the United States, 8.6% of adults have diabetes and 800,000 new cases of diabetes will be diagnosed in the upcoming year. Data from the National Health Interview Survey estimate that the lifetime risk of developing diabetes for

Table 1.2. Complications of Type 2 Diabetes

Acute Complications
- Diabetic ketoacidosis
- Hyperosmolar coma
- Hypoglycemia

Long-Term Complications

Microvascular
- Retinopathy
- Nephropathy
- Peripheral/autonomic neuropathy

Macrovascular
- Coronary heart disease
- Cerebrovascular disease
- Peripheral arterial disease

Other
- Decreased resistance to infection (with hyperglycemia)
- Skin changes
- Poor wound healing
- Cataracts
- Glaucoma
- Infertility
- Non-alcoholic steatosis/steatohepatitis (complication of insulin resistance)

individuals born in the U.S. in 2000 is 33% for men and 39% for females, resulting in large reductions in life expectancy and quality of life (JAMA 2003;290:1884-89). Stated another way, babies born in the US today have a one in three lifetime risk of developing diabetes and, if born into a high-risk ethnic group, the risk exceeds one in two. In addition, more than 5.5 million cases of diabetes in the U.S. are undiagnosed, and 26% of the American population (44% of those over age 60) have either impaired fasting glucose (prediabetes) or insulin resistance (metabolic syndrome), substantially increasing the risk of diabetes and cardiovascular events (Chapter 2). Elderly persons and certain ethnic groups (African Americans, Asians, Hispanics, Native Americans, Pacific Islanders) are at higher risk for developing diabetes. Today, 11% of American teenagers are prediabetic, and 10% of diabetes diagnosed in individuals under age 18 is type 2. In high-risk ethnic groups, as much as 50% of diabetes developing under age 18 is type 2 diabetes. The increasing prevalence of diabetes has been attributed to an aging population, increasing rates of obesity, declining levels of physical activity, and a high-carbohydrate, calorie dense diet consisting mostly of processed synthetic foods.

C. **Classification of Diabetes (Table 1.3)**

1. **Type 1 Diabetes.** This form of diabetes accounts for 5-10% of all cases. The vast majority of type 1 diabetes is caused by cell-mediated autoimmune destruction of the pancreatic islet beta-cells, resulting in failure of the pancreas to produce insulin and an absolute insulin deficiency. A family history of diabetes is less common than with type 2 diabetes. Twin studies show that 30-50% of the initially non-affected monozygotic twins will develop type 1 diabetes. Autoantibodies to islet cells, glutamic acid decarboxylase (GAD) and insulin are often present, and the risk for other autoimmune diseases is increased (Graves disease, Hashimoto's thyroiditis, Addison's disease, pernicious anemia). A small minority of cases are idiopathic (not autoimmune) in origin. Type 1 diabetes usually presents with the acute onset of symptoms (polyuria, polydipsia, polyphagia, weight loss) and disproportionately affects young people (70% of cases occur by age 20, though it can occur at any age), the majority of whom are not obese. Life-long insulin therapy is required for survival. Persons with type 1 diabetes are prone to diabetic ketoacidosis (DKA) because of an absolute deficiency of endogenous insulin, and DKA may be the initial manifestation of their disease. The terms "insulin dependent diabetes mellitus (IDDM)," "type I diabetes" (using the Roman numeral), and "juvenile onset diabetes mellitus" are no longer used to describe this condition.

2. **Type 2 Diabetes.** This form of diabetes accounts for 90-95% of all cases. Type 2 diabetes is caused by insulin resistance combined with an inability of the pancreatic beta cells to produce sufficient insulin to overcome the insulin resistance. Affected individuals almost always have a family history, particularly on the maternal side, probably due to a defect in the cofactor for the PPAR-gamma receptor in the mitochondria; this genetic predisposition in conjunction with behavioral and environmental risk factors—advanced age, obesity, and sedentary lifestyle—are responsible for

Table 1.3. Etiologic Classification of Diabetes Mellitus

Type 1 diabetes†*
- Immune-mediated (vast majority)
- Idiopathic

Type 2 diabetes‡*

Other specific types
- Genetic defects of beta-cell function or insulin action
- Diseases of the exocrine pancreas (pancreatitis, trauma/pancreatectomy, neoplasia, cystic fibrosis, hemochromatosis, fibrocalculous pancreatopathy)
- Endocrinopathies (acromegaly, Cushing's syndrome, glucagonoma, pheochromocytoma, hyperthyroidism, somatostatinoma, aldosteronoma, others)
- Drug- or chemical-induced (pentamidine, nicotinic acid, glucocorticoids, thyroid hormone, diazoxide, beta-adrenergic agonists, thiazides, dilantin, alpha-interferon, others)
- Infections (congenital rubella, cytomegalovirus, Coxsackie B, others)
- Uncommon forms of immune-mediated diabetes ("Stiff-man" syndrome, anti-insulin receptor antibodies, others)
- Other genetic syndromes sometimes associated with diabetes (Down's syndrome, Klinefelter's syndrome, Turner's syndrome, Wolfram's syndrome, Friedreich's ataxia, Huntington's chorea, Laurence-Moon-Biedl syndrome, myotonic dystrophy, porphyria, Prader-Willi syndrome, others)

Gestational diabetes mellitus (GDM)

† Beta cell destruction usually resulting in absolute insulin deficiency

‡ May range from predominantly insulin resistance with relative insulin deficiency to a predominantly secretory defect with insulin resistance

* Patients with any form of diabetes may require insulin treatment at some stage of their disease. Use of insulin does not, by itself, classify the patient.

From: The Expert Committee on the Diagnosis and Classification of Diabetes Mellitus, from the American Diabetes Association. Diabetes Care 2007;30(suppl 1):S4-S41.

the development of insulin resistance and diabetes. If one monozygotic twin develops type 2 diabetes, then over 90% of the initially non-affected twins will also develop the disease. In contrast to type 1 diabetes, type 2 diabetes historically affects people over the age of 40 (but is now seen as young as 3 years old), many of whom are obese, and autoimmune destruction of pancreatic islet beta cells does not occur. Less than one-third of type 2 diabetic patients will ultimately require insulin therapy, and episodes of spontaneous DKA are rare, but may develop during extreme stress or severe illness (Table 1.4), particularly in African Americans and Latinos. Importantly, early symptoms (fatigue, postprandial hypoglycemia) are often overlooked or ignored, and type 2 diabetes can go undetected for years, only to first present with a cardiovascular/neurological complication (e.g., MI, stroke, loss of vision, peripheral neuropathy). Diet, exercise, and weight loss can improve insulin resistance and occasionally appear to reverse type 2 diabetes in some obese people. Following bariatric surgery, increased GLP-1 production stimulates growth and suppresses apoptosis (programmed cell death) of insulin-producing beta cells, resulting in rates of recovery from diabetes of up to 75%. The term "non-insulin dependent diabetes mellitus (NIDDM)" is no longer used to describe this condition.

3. **Gestational Diabetes.** Gestational diabetes is defined as glucose intolerance that is first identified during pregnancy. The definition applies regardless of whether insulin or only diet modification is used for treatment or whether the condition persists after pregnancy. It does not exclude the possibility that unrecognized glucose intolerance may have antedated or started concomitantly with the pregnancy or that type 1 diabetes may develop during pregnancy. In the U.S., approximately 7% of all pregnancies are complicated by gestational diabetes, usually during the second or third trimester of pregnancy when elevated levels of human placental lactogen (HPL) raise insulin resistance. Hyperglycemia may be mild and asymptomatic, but treatment with insulin is often required to prevent fetal morbidity and mortality. Glucose tolerance typically reverts toward normal postpartum, but 35% of women are subsequently diagnosed with type 2 diabetes within 5-10 years. Pregnancy provides a "stress test" for the pancreas with suboptimal insulin secretion and warns that unless preventive measures are initiated the risk of type 2 diabetes in later life will be greatly increased.

4. **Other Types of Diabetes.** This category includes diabetes caused by genetic defects in beta-cell function or insulin action, genetic mitochondrial defects (maternal inherited diabetes mellitus plus deafness), diseases of the exocrine pancreas (e.g., hemochromatosis),

Table 1.4. Clinical Features of Diabetes Mellitus

	Type 1 Diabetes	Type 2 Diabetes
Prevalence (US)	0.4%	8.6%
Primary defect	Autoimmune (common) or idiopathic (rare) destruction of pancreatic islet beta-cells; insulin deficiency is usually absolute	Genetic, environmental factors resulting in insulin resistance with a combined insulin secretory defect; insulin deficiency is relative
Presentation	Acute onset of symptoms (polyuria, polydipsia, polyphagia, weight loss); often acutely ill; may present with ketoacidosis. Diagnosis is made soon after symptoms develop. Age at presentation < 20 years in 70% of cases; most are not obese	Subtle symptoms may go unnoticed/undetected for years. Vascular complication or neuropathy can be presenting complaint. Age at presentation is typically > 45 years; most are obese. Ketoacidosis is rare but may occur during severe illness/stress
Treatment	Insulin is required for survival. Hypoglycemia occurs more often in type 1 diabetes	Diet and exercise are sufficient in some and may reverse the condition. Most require oral drug therapy, and many require more than one agent. Insulin is eventually required in many

endocrinopathies (e.g., Cushing's syndrome, hyperthyroidism), drug/chemical-induced diabetes, and other conditions (Table 1.3).

5. **Other Disorders of Glucose Regulation.** Impaired glucose tolerance (IGT) and impaired fasting glucose (IFG) are risk factors for diabetes. These conditions are also referred to as "prediabetes," as 25% of affected individuals eventually develop type 2 diabetes. All persons with IGT or IFG should receive instruction on therapeutic lifestyle changes (Chapter 4). A fasting plasma glucose is recommended

annually to detect the onset of diabetes and the need for more aggressive therapy. Several interventions have been shown to reduce the progression from prediabetes to diabetes, including diet/exercise (58% reduction), rosiglitazone (60% reduction), metformin (31% reduction), acarbose (25% reduction), and bariatric surgery (70% reduction) (Chapter 2). Studies are in progress (e.g., NAVIGATOR [ARB and nateglinide], ACT NOW [pioglitazone]) to determine whether other pharmacological interventions can prevent or delay the development of type 2 diabetes.

D. Presentation. The most common presentation of type 1 diabetes is polyuria with polydipsia. Other symptoms include weight loss despite increased appetite, blurred vision, drowsiness, poor stamina, nausea, frequent skin and bladder infections, and Candida vaginitis in women. In type 1 diabetes, symptoms usually develop abruptly over weeks, and patients may be acutely ill on presentation. In type 2 diabetes, symptoms may gradually appear over months to years, making this condition easy to overlook or ignore, and patients often do not recognize that they are unwell until a dramatic improvement in "well being" occurs with diabetic therapy. Reactive hypoglycemia due to a loss of first-phase insulin response, post-prandial hyperglycemia, and hyperinsulinemia leading to late hypoglycemia are often present early in the course of type 2 diabetes. Chronic and undiagnosed hyperglycemia in type 2 diabetes can induce pathological changes in organ tissues before symptoms are recognized, and at the time of diagnosis of diabetes, a microvascular or neurologic complication is present in 20% of patients. Occasionally, the initial manifestation of diabetes is a vascular complication (retinopathy, nephropathy, MI, stroke, heart failure), peripheral neuropathy, or a medical emergency that can threaten survival without hospitalization and treatment (DKA, nonketotic hyperosmolar coma). Approximately two-thirds of subjects presenting with stable CHD or acute coronary syndrome have either type 2 diabetes or impaired glucose tolerance (Am J Cardiol 2005;96:363-5). In patients who do not have diabetes at the time of their first MI, over the next 5 years the risk of developing type 2 diabetes is increased 2-3–fold in men and 3-4–fold in women (Diabet Med 2005;22:1334-7).

E. **Screening for Diabetes.** Many diabetic individuals are asymptomatic and can go undiagnosed for years, during which time pathological changes can develop in non-insulin sensitive tissues due to exposure to hyperglycemia. Early diagnosis and treatment of type 2 diabetes can prevent the development of microvascular and macrovascular complications. Therefore, the American Diabetes Association recommends screening all high-risk individuals for diabetes (Table 1.5).

F. **Diagnosis (Table 1.6).** The American Diabetes Association requires the presence of one of the following criteria for the diagnosis of diabetes (Diabetes Care 2006;29[suppl 1]:S4-S42):
- Unequivocal elevation of plasma glucose concentrations on more than one occasion associated with classic symptoms of diabetes
- Elevation of fasting plasma glucose (FPG) on more than one occasion
- Elevation of plasma glucose following a standardized oral glucose tolerance test

G. **Management of Diabetes.** Traditional therapeutic efforts aimed predominantly at normalizing elevated glucose levels without aggressively controlling other modifiable risk factors associated with insulin resistance have proven inadequate for reducing cardiovascular events in type 2 diabetes. Optimal management requires a coordinated team approach aimed at intensive glycemic control, improving insulin sensitivity, treatment of dyslipidemia and hypertension, management of diabetes-related complications, and patient education.

H. **Natural History and Prognosis.** Type 2 diabetes is a chronic, progressive disorder resulting in gradual loss of pancreatic islet beta cell function and the need for escalating drug therapy over time. If left unchecked, rising HbA_{1c} levels increase the risk of microvascular and macrovascular complications. The lifetime risk of developing diabetes for individuals born in the U.S. today is one in three, and the presence of diabetes markedly reduces both long-term survival and quality of life. (For diabetes diagnosed at age 40, long-term survival and quality of survival are reduced by approximately 12.5 years and 20 years, respectively [JAMA 2003;290:1884-1889]). Preventive strategies can delay the onset/slow the progression of diabetes-related complications (Chapters 2, 6-9).

Table 1.5. Screening for Diabetes in Asymptomatic Individuals*

Testing should be considered for age ≥ 45 years, particularly in those with a BMI ≥ 25 kg/m²†. If the test is normal, it should be repeated at 3-year intervals.
Testing should be considered at a younger age or be carried out more frequently in overweight (BMI ≥ 25 kg/m²†) individuals with additional risk factors:

- first-degree relative with diabetes
- habitually physically inactive
- member of a high-risk ethnic population (e.g., African American, Hispanic American, Native American, Asian American, Pacific Islander)
- delivery of a baby weighing > 9 lbs or history of gestational diabetes
- hypertension (BP ≥ 140/90 mmHg)
- HDL cholesterol ≤ 35 mg/dL or triglyceride ≥ 250 mg/dL
- polycystic ovary syndrome
- impaired glucose tolerance or impaired fasting glucose on previous testing
- history of vascular disease

* Fasting plasma glucose or an oral glucose tolerance test may be used to diagnose diabetes (Table 1.6).

† May not be correct for all ethnic groups

From: Standards of Medical Care in Diabetes. The American Diabetes Association. Diabetes Care 2007;30(suppl 1):S4-S41.

Table 1.6. Criteria for the Diagnosis of Diabetes Mellitus

Category	Fasting Plasma Glucose (mg/dL)	2-Hour Plasma Glucose† (mg/dL)	Casual Plasma Glucose†† (mg/dL)
Normoglycemia	< 100	< 140	–
IFG/IGT	100-125 / –	– / 140-199	–
Diabetes	≥ 126*	≥ 200	> 200 with symptoms of diabetes*

IFG = impaired fasting glucose, IGT = impaired glucose tolerance

* A diagnosis of diabetes must be confirmed on a subsequent day. The fasting plasma glucose test is preferred because of ease of administration, convenience, acceptability to patients, and lower cost. Fasting is defined as no caloric intake for at least 8 hours.

† This test requires the use of a glucose load containing the equivalent of 75 gm anhydrous glucose in water followed by plasma glucose measurement 2 hours later

†† Anytime of day without regard to last meal

From: The American Diabetes Association. Diabetes Care 2007;30(suppl 1):S42-S47.

Chapter 2

Metabolic Syndrome, Insulin Resistance, Prediabetes, and Prevention of Type 2 Diabetes

A. **The Metabolic Syndrome.** The metabolic syndrome is characterized by a cluster of metabolic abnormalities that increases cardiovascular risk, chief among them being insulin resistance. Approximately 24% (47 million) of adult Americans have the metabolic syndrome, and the prevalence of this disorder is escalating. The diagnosis requires the presence of at least 3 of 5 major criteria, as defined by the National Cholesterol Education Program Adult Treatment Panel III (Table 2.1). Individuals with the metabolic syndrome are at increased risk of developing diabetes and cardiovascular events, the latter due to accelerated atherosclerosis, hypercoagulability, and endothelial dysfunction (Table 2.2). Compared to men without any of the 5 features of the metabolic syndrome, those with 4 or 5 features have a 25-fold increased risk of new diabetes and a 4-fold increased risk of coronary heart disease; the presence of inflammation, manifest as elevated C-reactive protein, further increases risk (Circulation 2003;108:414-419). Environmental factors, such as excessive saturated fat, processed carbohydrate and calorie intake; obesity; and sedentary lifestyle substantially increase the risk of developing the metabolic syndrome and

Table 2.1. Criteria for the Diagnosis of the Metabolic Syndrome*

- Abdominal obesity: waist circumference > 102 cm (40 in) in men or > 88 cm (35 in) in women
- Triglycerides ≥ 150 mg/dL
- HDL cholesterol < 40 mg/dL in men or < 50 mg/dL in women
- Blood pressure ≥ 130/85 mmHg
- Impaired fasting glucose (fasting glucose 100-125 mg/dL)

* Clinical identification of the metabolic syndrome requires the presence of at least 3 of 5 factors. The metabolic syndrome is associated with an increased risk of new diabetes and cardiovascular events. From: Circulation 2004;109:433-438.

Table 2.2. Pathophysiological Changes Associated with the Metabolic Syndrome

Some degree of glucose intolerance

- Impaired fasting glucose: plasma glucose 100-125 mg/dL
- Impaired glucose intolerance: plasma glucose 140-199 mg/dL 2 hours after a 75-gram oral glucose challenge

Dyslipidemia

- Triglycerides > 150 mg/dL
- HDL cholesterol < 40 mg/dL (men), < 50 mg/dL (women)
- Increased small, dense, atherogenic LDL and ApoB particles
- Postprandial elevation of triglyceride-rich lipoproteins

Endothelial dysfunction

- Increased mononuclear cell adhesion
- Elevated plasma concentration of cellular adhesion molecules
- Impaired endothelial-dependent vasodilatation

Hemodynamic changes

- Augmented sympathetic nervous system activity
- Renal sodium retention
- Elevated blood pressure

Prothrombotic factors

- Increased plasminogen activator inhibitor-1
- Increased fibrinogen

Inflammation

- Increased C-reactive protein, white blood cells, etc.

Increased plasma uric acid concentration

These changes increase the risk of cardiovascular disease

type 2 diabetes. (Decades ago, diabetes was rare in the Inuit population, who followed a traditional hunter-gatherer lifestyle of extensive daily physical exertion. Today, after developing a more sedentary lifestyle and embracing a Westernized diet of increased calories, processed carbohydrates, and trans fats, approximately 75% of Inuits are obese and 66% of Inuit women have type 2 diabetes.) Genetics also impact insulin sensitivity—offspring of individuals with type 2 diabetes, hypertension, or atherosclerosis have higher degrees of insulin resistance than offspring of healthy controls. With aging, mitochondrial function declines and insulin resistance worsens.

The problem with the ATP III definition is lack of ethnic specific criteria for obesity. The International Diabetes Federation (IDF) recommended a new definition with a goal of emphasizing the role of central obesity and insulin resistance as causative factors. They recommended that the waist circumference plus any two additional factors, using the same metabolic criteria, be required to make the diagnosis of metabolic syndrome. Additionally, they created ethnic specific criteria for the measurement of waist circumference and recommended that ethnic group specific cut-points should be used for people of the same ethnic group regardless of where the person lives. This new definition still needs to undergo peer review but should allow identification of the metabolic syndrome in ethnic groups who are insulin resistant at lower BMIs than the general US population. In clinical practice, if the triglyceride-to-HDL ratio is greater than 3.5, then it is likely that the patient has insulin resistance and is at increased risk for cardiovascular disease and diabetes (Am J Cardiol 2005;96;399-404).

Research has now shown that in some individuals the genetic defect is a defect of PPG-1, a coactivator of the PPAR-gamma receptor in the mitochondria (N Eng J Med 2004;350:664-71). Treatment of the metabolic syndrome requires increased physical activity (Chapter 4), weight control (Chapter 4), and optimal management of hypertension and dyslipidemia (Chapters 7-8). The American College of Endocrinology has recommended that persons with the metabolic syndrome be treated to the same LDL target as those with diabetes (< 100 mg/dL). Diet modification, smoking cessation, and use of antiplatelet therapy and ACE inhibitors for high risk individuals are also indicated for overall cardiovascular health (Chapters 4, 9).

B. Insulin Resistance, Hyperinsulinemia, and Cardiovascular Disease. Insulin resistance is the underlying pathophysiological defect in both the metabolic syndrome and type 2 diabetes. Characterized by marked impairment of insulin-stimulated glucose uptake by peripheral tissues, insulin resistance is associated with increases in free fatty acid production, hepatic glucose production, insulin levels, and the risk of

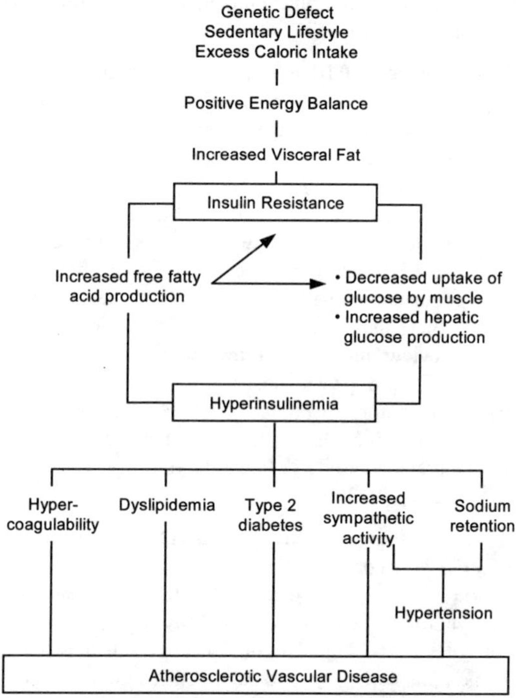

Figure 2.1. Insulin Resistance, Hyperinsulinemia, and Atherosclerosis

Sedentary lifestyle, poor diet, and obesity lead to insulin resistance, hyperinsulinemia, and increased risk of cardiovascular events.

atherosclerotic vascular disease (Figure 2.1). Approximately 30% of the American population have insulin resistance, including 58% of persons with hypertension, 65% with coronary disease, and 85% with hypertriglyceridemia or low HDL cholesterol. Compared to persons with normal glucose homeostasis, insulin-resistant individuals with hyperinsulinemia or impaired fasting glucose are at increased risk of

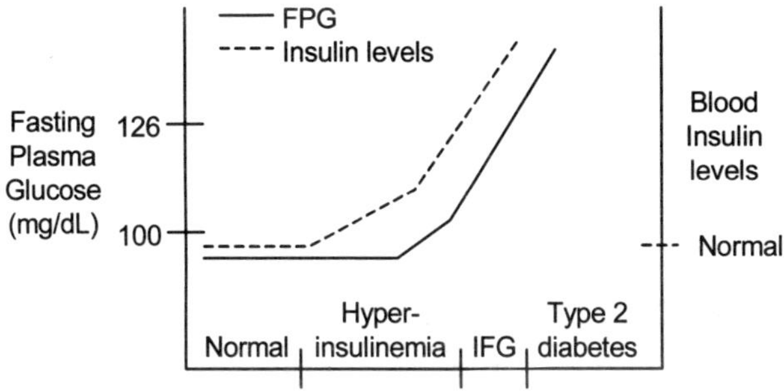

Figure 2.2. Insulin Levels and Glycemia in Type 2 Diabetes

As muscle becomes more resistant to insulin, increased insulin levels are required to maintain normal plasma glucose levels. Over time, elevated insulin levels are unable to keep pace with progressive insulin resistance, resulting in impaired fasting glucose (IFG). Insulin-resistant individuals often develop a cluster of cardiovascular risk factors (metabolic syndrome) that increases the risk of cardiac death, MI, and stroke (Table 2.2). Insulin levels may remain elevated early in type 2 diabetes but eventually decline due to loss of beta cell function (Figure 2.4). The "ticking clock" hypothesis states that atherosclerosis and increased risk of adverse events begin when insulin resistance develops, typically years to decades before type 2 diabetes is diagnosed.

cardiovascular events (Figures 2.2, 2.3). The risk of non-alcoholic fatty liver disease, polycystic ovarian syndrome, and possibly several forms of cancer (e.g., breast) are increased as well. Insulin resistance is treated the same as the metabolic syndrome, with emphasis placed on improving insulin sensitivity through weight control and increased physical activity. Weight loss by as little as 5-15% of body weight in overweight/obese individuals with insulin resistance can substantially improve insulin sensitivity, reduce plasma glucose levels, and improve manifestations of the metabolic syndrome. Substantial weight loss, as achieved with gastric bypass, results in normoglycemia for a sustained period in approximately

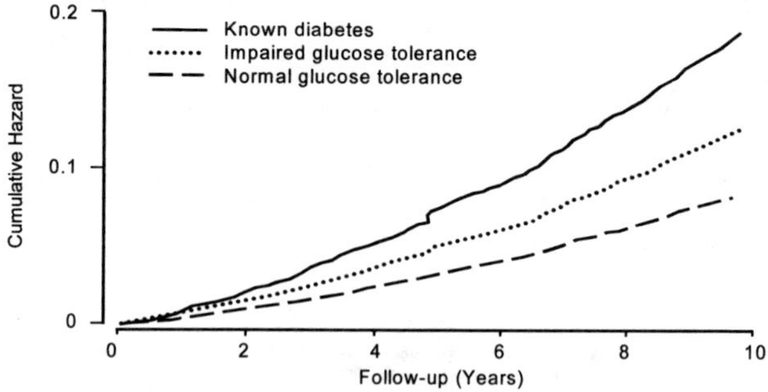

Figure 2.3. Insulin Resistance and Cardiovascular Risk

This risk of cardiovascular disease increases with the development of insulin resistance and hyperinsulinemia. Individuals with impaired glucose tolerance or the metabolic syndrome have cardiovascular risk that is intermediate between normal subjects and those with type 2 diabetes. From: Lancet 1999;354:617-621.

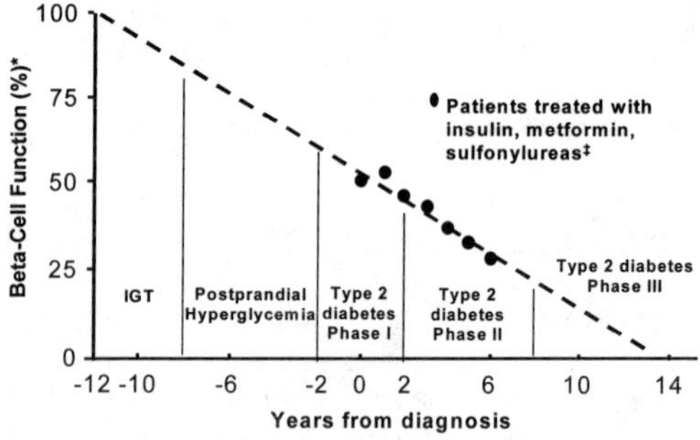

Figure 2.4. Loss of Pancreatic Beta Cell Function in UKPDS

IGT = impaired glucose tolerance. Typically, up to 50% of beta cell function has been lost by the time type 2 diabetes is diagnosed. After 15 years of diabetes, less than 10% of beta cells are functioning and insulin replacement therapy is often required.

* Dashed line shows extrapolation forward and backward from years 0-6 from diagnosis of diabetes based on Homeostasis Model Assessment data from UKPDS.

From: Diabetes Rev 1999;7:139-153.

70%, though this may be due to improved beta cell function (see Chapter 5). Evolving evidence suggests that a low-glycemic load, high fiber diet with adequate amounts of monounsaturated and omega-3 fats and lean protein can improve satiety, dietary thermogenesis (basal metabolic rate), and insulin sensitivity. Non-fat dairy products, soy foods, and modest alcohol intake (not more than 1 drink per day in women or 2 drinks per day in men) can also improve insulin sensitivity (Table 2.3). Exercise lowers glucose levels acutely and for up to 48 hours after physical activity, lowers triglyceride levels, raises HDL levels, and facilitates weight loss. Among oral diabetic medications, thiazolidinediones (TZD's) directly improve insulin resistance. Other agents may indirectly improve insulin resistance by lowering glucose, and metformin improves insulin resistance by reducing food intake and body weight.

Table 2.3. Effect of Dietary Modifications on Insulin Resistance

Improves Insulin Resistance	Worsens Insulin Resistance
Decreased caloric intake	High-glycemic load foods
Minimally-processed vegetables, fruits, legumes, and whole grains	Trans fats and saturated fats
Fiber	Excess calorie intake
Lean protein	Highly-processed, easily digested foods
Light-to-moderate alcohol intake	
Nuts	
Non-fat dairy	
Cinnamon	

C. **Importance of Postprandial Hyperglycemia on Cardiovascular Risk Factors, Atherosclerosis, and Cardiac Events.** Epidemiological data consistently demonstrate that postprandial hyperglycemia is an independent predictor of future cardiovascular events in diabetic and nondiabetic subjects (Figure 2.5). The cardiovascular toxicity of postprandial hyperglycemia appears to be mediated by oxidant stress, which is directly proportional to glucose and lipid excursion after a meal. This transient increase in free radical formation acutely triggers inflammation, endothelial dysfunction, hypercoagulability, sympathetic hyperactivity, and a cascade of other atherogenic changes (Figure 2.6). Early studies found that blunting of postprandial spikes in plasma glucose led to an immediate reduction in vascular inflammation and improved endothelial function. Recent randomized controlled trials suggest that improving postprandial dysmetabolism may also reduce the incidence of type 2 diabetes (DREAM trial) and hypertension (STOP-NIDDM trial) and slow the progression of atherosclerosis (Figure 2.7). Measures shown to improve postprandial hyperglycemia include diet/exercise (also improves postprandial lipids), exenatide, rosiglitazone, pioglitazone, acarbose, nateglinide, repaglinide, ultra–fast-acting insulins, inhaled insulin, and DPP-4 inhibitors.

D. **Prevention of Type 2 Diabetes.** The incidence of diabetes and prediabetes has been on a steeply rising trajectory that parallels the obesity epidemic. More than 150 million people worldwide have diabetes, and the number of cases is expected to double by the year 2025. The typical American born today has a one in three chance of developing type 2 diabetes; for Hispanics and African-Americans, the risk is one in two. Diabetes confers a level of cardiovascular risk similar to that associated with a history of prior MI and is considered a "CHD risk equivalent." (The converse is also true: over 70% of people who present with CHD have abnormal glucose metabolism [European Heart Journal 2004;25:1880-1890].) Risk factors for the development of type 2 diabetes are shown in Table 2.4. For a male diagnosed with diabetes at age 40, average life expectancy is reduced by approximately 12.5 years and quality of life by 20 years (JAMA 2003;290:1884-90). Because of its high prevalence and grave health consequences, the prevention of type 2 diabetes has become a major focus of health care. Diet and exercise can substantially improve insulin sensitivity, lower plasma insulin levels, improve manifestations of the metabolic syndrome, and prevent/delay type 2 diabetes by up to 58%. Rosiglitazone, metformin, acarbose, troglitazone, and orlistat have also been shown to reduce new diabetes in prospective randomized trials (Table 2.5). The largest and most impressive of these studies was the Diabetes REduction Assessment with ramipril and rosiglitazone Medication (DREAM) trial, which evaluated the effectiveness of rosiglitazone and/or ramipril for preventing type 2 diabetes and death in prediabetic individuals. A total of 5269 adults aged 30 years or more with IFG (mean FPG 104 mg/dL) or IGT (mean 2-hour

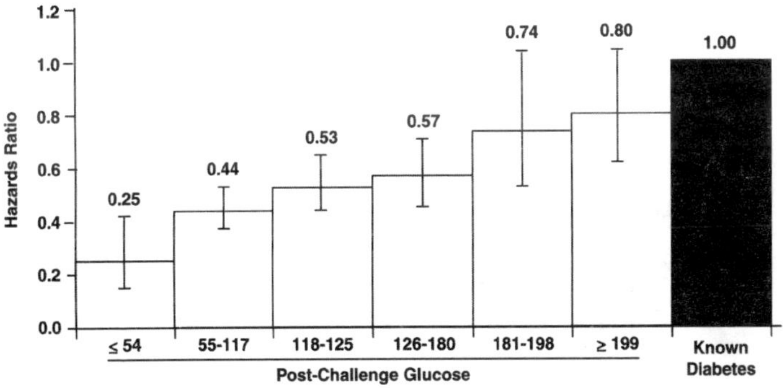

Figure 2.5. Postprandial Glucose Levels and Cardiovascular Risk

The risk of cardiovascular death increases 300% as 2-hour post-challenge glucose levels rise from 54 mg/dL to 200 mg/dL, despite the fact that these readings are all in the nondiabetic range. Hazard ratios and 95% confidence intervals for cardiovascular mortality, as assessed during 11-year follow up for 29,714 patients in the DECODE study. From: Diabetes Care 2003; 26:688-96.

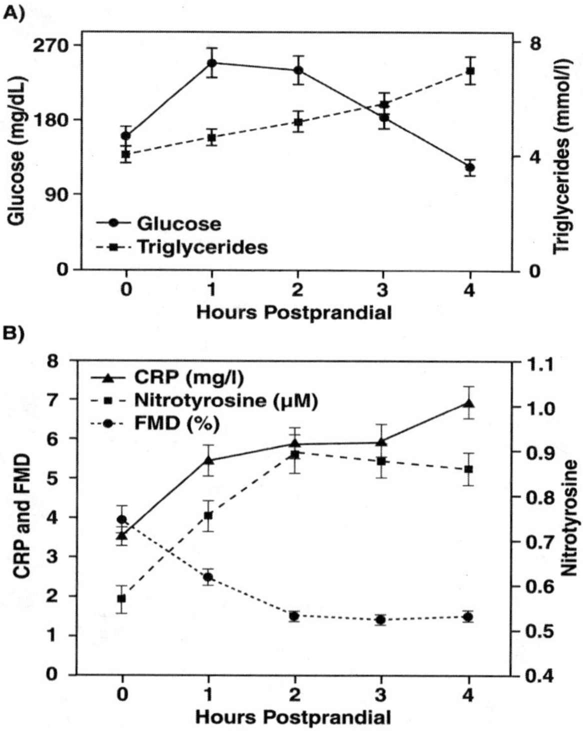

Figure 2.6. Postprandial Glucose Levels and Endothelial Function

The immediate deleterious effects of a meal containing 75 grams of glucose and 700 kcal/m^2 of whipping cream in 20 diabetic subjects. (A) Within 2-4 hours glucose and triglyceride levels double. (B) This causes immediate oxidant stress (increased nitrotyrosine levels) and vascular inflammation (increased CRP), resulting in deterioration in endothelial function (reduction in percent flow mediated dilatation, FMD). From: Circulation 2005;111:2518-24.

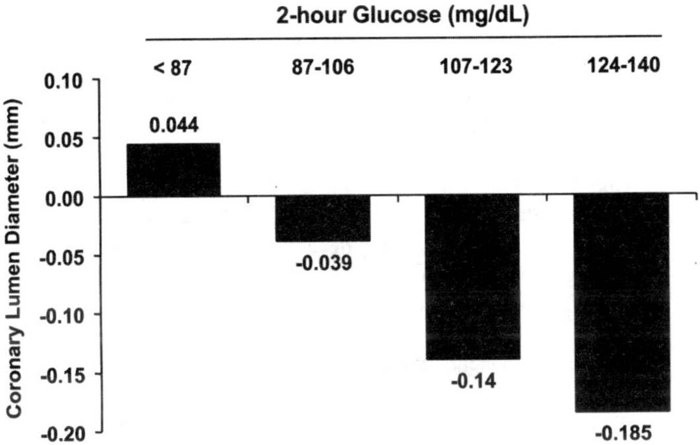

Figure 2.7. Postprandial Glucose Levels and Progression of Atherosclerosis

Angiographic coronary disease progression as measured by change in minimum coronary lumen diameter. In this cohort of patients with normal glucose tolerance as defined by a 2-hour postchallenge glucose of < 140mg/dL, the patients who showed a peak postprandial glucose of less that 87 mg/dL had coronary regression. The remaining patients had coronary progression in proportion to the rise in postprandial glucose. From: Arterioscler Thromb Vasc Biol 2006;26:189-93.

post-challenge blood glucose 156 mg/dL) were randomized to rosiglitazone 8 mg/d or placebo in a factorial design. After three years, rosiglitazone reduced the primary endpoint—new diabetes or death—by 60% (11.6% of the rosiglitazone group versus 26.0% of the placebo group, $p < 0.0001$) (Figure 2.8). Additionally, 50.5% of rosiglitazone-treated patients versus 30.3% of the placebo group reverted back to normoglycemia during the course of the study ($p < 0.0001$). Cardiovascular event rates were similar in the two groups, except for congestive heart failure, which developed in 0.5% of the rosiglitazone group and in 0.1% of the placebo group ($p = 0.01$). At study end, the median fasting plasma glucose was 9 mg/dL lower and the 2-hour post-challenge blood glucose was 30 mg/dL lower in the rosiglitazone group compared to placebo. Based on these results it was estimated that rosiglitazone 8 mg/d for 3 years would prevent one in every seven people with IGT or IFG from developing diabetes (Lancet 2006;368:1096-1105). Several other large trials suggest that ACE inhibitors, angiotensin receptor blockers (ARB's) and rimonobant may also be useful in preventing new diabetes (Table 2.6). In a meta-analysis of post-hoc analyses of 13 randomized ACE inhibitor and ARB trials, including 90,474 patients without diabetes at baseline, risk reduction for new onset diabetes was 24% for ACE inhibitors and 23% for ARBs (overall RRR 0.77 [95% CI: 0.71-0.83]) (J Am Coll Cardiol 2005;46:821-826). The new diagnosis of diabetes was a prespecified endpoint in the VALUE trial, which compared the blood pressure effects of valsartan (ARB) versus amlodipine, a calcium channel blocker. A 23% decrease in new onset diabetes was seen in the valsartan treated group. In contrast, simvastatin did not reduce the prespecified endpoint of new-onset diabetes in the Heart Protection Study (HPS) megatrial. Additional trials will be needed to confirm these findings, and other prospective trials are underway (NAVIGATOR: valsartan and nateglinide; ONTARGET: ramipril and telmisartan; ACT NOW: pioglitazone). At present, no pharmacologic agent is approved for the prevention of diabetes.

Table 2.4. Risk Factors for Type 2 Diabetes

- Age ≥ 45 years
- Overweight (body mass index ≥ 25 kg/m^2*)
- First-degree relative with diabetes
- Habitual physical inactivity
- Member of a high-risk ethnic population (e.g., African American, Latino, Native American, Asian American, Pacific Islander)
- Impaired fasting glucose (IFG) or impaired glucose tolerance (IGT)
- History of gestational diabetes or delivery of a baby weighting > 9 lbs
- Hypertensive (≥ 140/90 mmHg)
- HDL cholesterol ≤ 35 mg/dL or triglyceride level ≥ 250 mg/dL
- Polycystic ovary syndrome
- History of vascular disease

* May not be correct for all ethnic groups. From: Diabetes Care 2007;30(suppl 1)

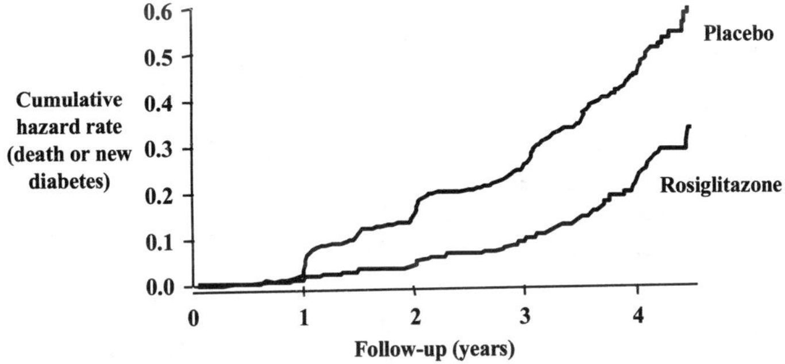

Figure 2.8. Results of the DREAM Trial

Rosiglitazone 8 mg/d for 3 years reduced by 60% the incidence of new diabetes in adults with impaired fasting glucose (IFG) or impaired glucose tolerance (IGT) (11.6% in the rosiglitazone group vs. 26% in the placebo group, RRR 60%, HR 0.40 [0.35-0.46], $p < 0.0001$). Reversion to normoglycemia was also significantly more likely to occur with rosiglitazone ($p < 0.0001$). From: Lancet 2006; 268:1096-1105.

Table 2.5. Prevention of Type 2 Diabetes: Randomized Controlled Trials in Persons with Impaired Glucose Tolerance (IGT)

Trial	No. Patients	Follow-up (years)	Risk Reduction Measure	Reduction in New Diabetes
DREAM	5269	3	Rosiglitazone Ramipril	60% 9%
Diabetes Prevention Project (DPP)	3234	2.8	Metformin Lifestyle change	31% 58%
Indian Diabetes Prevention Program	531	2.5	Metformin Lifestyle change	26% 29%
Finish Diabetes Prevention Study	522	3.2	Intensive lifestyle change	58%
Da Quing IGT & Diabetes Study	577	6	Diet and/or exercise	31-46%
SOS	1703	10	Bariatric surgery	70%
STOP-NIDDM	1400	3.9	Acarbose	25%
TRIPOD	266*	2.5	Troglitazone	55%
XENDOS	3304	4	Orlistat	37%

* Hispanic women with gestational diabetes mellitus

Lifestyle changes are recommended for all patients at risk for developing type 2 diabetes. No drug therapy has been approved for the prevention of new diabetes. References: DREAM: Diabetes Reduction Assessment with Ramipril and Rosiglitazone Medication (Lancet 2006;368:1096-1105); DPP: Diabetes Prevention Study (N Engl J Med 2001;344:1343-1350); Indian Diabetes Prevention Study (Diabetologia 2006;49:289-97); SOS: Swedish Obese Subjects (N Eng J Med 2004;351:2683-93); STOP-NIDDM: Study to Prevent NIDDM (Lancet 2002;359:2072-2077); TRIPOD: Troglitazone in the Prevention of Diabetes (Diabetes 2002;51:2796-2803); XENDOS: Xenical in the Prevention of Diabetes in Obese Subjects (Rev Med Liege 2002;57:617-621).

Table 2.6. Prevention of Type 2 Diabetes: Other Randomized Trials†

Trial	No. Patients	Follow-up (years)	Comparison	Reduction in New Diabetes
VALUE	15,245 with hypertension + ASVD or diabetes	4.2	Valsartan vs. amlodipine	23%
HOPE	9297 with ASVD or diabetes*	5	Ramipril vs. placebo	34%
ALLHAT	24,309 with hypertension + 1 cardiac risk factor	4.9	Lisinopril vs. chlorthalidone	30%
PEACE	8290 with CHD	4.8	Trandolapril vs. placebo	20%
ANBP2	6083 with hypertension	4.1	Enalapril vs. hydrochlorothiazide	33%
CAPPP	10,985 with hypertension	5	Captopril vs. diuretic/beta-blocker	15%
ASCOT	19,257 with hypertension plus ≥ 3 other risk factors	5.4	Amlodipine/ perindopril vs. atenolol/diuretic	32%
LIFE	9193 with hypertension/ LVH	4.8	Losartan vs. atenolol	25%
CHARM	7601 with chronic heart failure	3.2	Candesartan vs. placebo	29%
COMET	3029 with chronic heart failure	4.8	Carvedilol vs. metoprolol	22%

ASVD = atherosclerotic vascular disease, LVH = left ventricular hypertrophy

† All are post-hoc analyses except for VALUE, where prevention of new diabetes was a prespecified endpoint. No drug therapy approved for the prevention of new diabetes

* With at least 1 other cardiovascular risk factor

References: VALUE (Lancet 2004;363:2022-31); HOPE (N Engl J Med 2000;342:145-153, JAMA 2001;286:1882-5); ALLHAT (JAMA 2002;288:2981-2997, JAMA 2000;283:1967-1975); PEACE (N Engl J Med 2004;251:2058-68); ANBP2 (N Engl J Med 2003;348:583-92); CAPPP (Lancet 1999;353:611-616, Diabetes Care 2001;24:2091-2096); ASCOT (ACC meeting, March, 2005, Orlando, FL); LIFE (Lancet 2002;359:995-1003); CHARM (Lancet 2003;362:759-766); COMET (Lancet 2003;362:7-13).

Chapter 3

Overview of Treatment of Type 2 Diabetes

Once the diagnosis of diabetes has been established (Chapter 1), the medical history, physical examination, and laboratory testing (Table 3.1) are used to identify cardiovascular risk factors and target organ damage:

- *Cardiovascular risk factors*: hypertension, dyslipidemia, sedentary lifestyle, overweight/obesity, tobacco use, atherogenic diet
- *Cardiovascular disease:* angina, prior MI or coronary revascularization, heart failure, left ventricular hypertrophy
- *Cerebrovascular disease:* carotid bruit, transient ischemic attack, stroke
- *Retinopathy:* microaneurysms, hard exudates, macular edema, soft exudates (retinal infarcts), neovascularization, vitreous hemorrhage, retinal detachment, macular ischemia
- *Nephropathy:* increased serum creatinine, micro/macroalbuminuria
- *Peripheral artery disease:* claudication, aneurysm, absence of peripheral pulses, foot ulcers, loss of hair growth, shiny thin skin
- *Neuropathy:* altered light touch/pain/vibration, orthostatic hypotension, gastroparesis, urinary retention, diabetic diarrhea, impotence, muscle weakness, neuropathic pain, foot ulcers, interosseous muscle wasting

Glycemic Control

Epidemiologic analysis from the United Kingdom Prospective Diabetes Study (UKPDS) Group demonstrated a continuous relationship between baseline glycemia and the risk of vascular complications: each 1% decrease in HbA_{1c} was associated with a 35% reduction in microvascular complications, a 25% reduction in diabetes-related deaths, an 18% reduction in MI, and a 7% reduction in all-cause mortality. Compared to patients treated conservatively with diet in UKPDS (mean HbA_{1c} 7.9%), intensive glycemic therapy with either a sulfonylurea or insulin (mean HbA_{1c} 7%) was

Table 3.1. Clinical Evaluation of Type 2 Diabetes

Medical History

- Symptoms, laboratory tests, other results related to the diagnosis of diabetes
- Prior HbA_{1c} records and details of previous and current treatment programs (medications, meal plan, results of glucose monitoring and patients' use of data)
- Eating patterns, nutritional status, and weight history; growth and development in children and adolescents; exercise history
- Frequency, severity, cause of acute complications (e.g., ketoacidosis, hypoglycemia)
- Prior or current infections (e.g., skin, foot, dental, genitourinary)
- Symptoms and treatment of complication of diabetes (eye, kidney, nerve, heart, peripheral vascular, bladder, GI, foot, cerebrovascular)
- Other medications that may affect blood glucose levels
- Risk factors for atherosclerosis (smoking, hypertension, overweight/obesity, dyslipidemia, sedentary lifestyle, family history)
- History and treatment of other conditions, including endocrine and eating disorders
- Family history of diabetes and other endocrine disorders
- Lifestyle, cultural, psychosocial, educational, and economic factors that might influence the management of diabetes
- Tobacco, alcohol, controlled substance use
- Contraception and reproductive/sexual history

Physical Examination

- Height, weight, waist circumference measurements
- Blood pressure (including orthostatic) measurements
- Funduscopic, oral, thyroid, cardiac, hand/finger examinations
- Neurological exam, including vibration sense (tuning fork)/fine sensation (monofilament)
- Abdominal examination (e.g., for hepatomegaly); skin examination (for acanthosis nigricans and insulin-injection sites); evaluation of pulses by palpation/auscultation
- Signs of diseases that can cause secondary diabetes (e.g., hemochromatosis, pancreatic disease, Cushing's disease)

Laboratory Evaluation

- HbA_{1c}
- Fasting total/LDL/HDL cholesterol and triglycerides
- Test for microalbuminuria; urinalysis for ketones, protein, sediment
- Serum creatinine in adults (in children if proteinuria is present)
- Thyroid-stimulating hormone (TSH) if clinically indicated
- Bone density in adults > 50 years old (diabetes is a risk factor for osteoporosis)
- Electrocardiogram in adults

Referrals

- Eye exam; family planning for women of reproductive age; diabetes educator, if not provided by physician or staff; behavioral specialist; foot specialist; dietician; others

Adapted from: The American Diabetes Association. Diabetes Care 2007;30(suppl 1):S4-S41.

associated with a highly significant 25% reduction in microvascular complications and a 16% reduction in MI and death at 10 years ($p = 0.052$). The Norfolk Epic Study showed that for each 1% HbA_{1c} increase above 5% and 7%, cardiac events increased by 26% and 40%, respectively.

A. **Goals of Therapy.** Diabetes treatment goals differ somewhat between the American Diabetes Association (ADA), the American Association of Clinical Endocrinologists/American College of Endocrinology (AACE/ACE), and the International Diabetes Federation (Table 3.2). (The ADA recommendation is based on the results of DCCT, a type 1 diabetes study [p. 146]; the AACE/ACE recommendation is based on the results of UKPDS, a type 2 study [p. 150]. In general, efforts should be made to reduce HbA_{1c} to the lowest possible level at which frequent or severe hypoglycemic episodes do not occur. Unlike patients with type 1

Table 3.2. Treatment Targets for Adults with Diabetes

	Normal§	ADA Target	AACE/ACE Target
Glycemic control			
HbA_{1c} (%)*	< 6.0	< 7.0	< 6.5
Plasma glucose			
preprandial	< 100	90-130	< 110
postprandial	< 140†	< 180¶	< 140†
Blood pressure (mmHg)	< 120/80	< 130/80	–
Lipids (mg/dL)			
LDL	Varies	< 100‡	–
Triglycerides‡	< 150	< 150‡	–
HDL	> 40	> 40	–

AACE/ACE = American Association of Clinical Endocrinologists/American College of Endocrinology (Endocr Pract 2002;8[suppl 1]:5-11), ADA = American Diabetes Association (Diabetes Care 2007;30[suppl 1]:S4-S41)

§ Normal levels in persons without diabetes

* Referenced to a nondiabetic range of 4.0-6.0% using a DCCT-based assay

† 2-hour postprandial

¶ Peak postprandial

‡ For diabetic patients with established CHD or other clinical forms of atherosclerosis, it is reasonable to treat to an optional LDL-C < 70 mg/dL and, if triglycerides ≥ 200 mg/dL, to an optional non–HDL-C < 100 mg/dL (Circulation 2004;110:227-239, Circulation 2006;113:2363-2372) (also see Chapter 7)

diabetes, in most patients with type 2 diabetes, HbA_{1c} levels between 6-7% are readily achieved. This is especially the case in the earlier stages of type 2 diabetes when endogenous insulin production is still high, particularly if drugs that do not cause hypoglycemia are utilized (metformin, TZD's, alpha-glucosidase inhibitors, DPP-4 inhibitors) (Chapter 5). The risks and benefits of treating patients with type 2 diabetes to a $HbA_{1c} < 6\%$ are under evaluation in the Action to Control Cardiovascular Risk in Diabetes (ACCORD) trial.

B. **Assessment of Glycemic Control.** Monitoring of glycemic status by patients and physicians is essential to diabetes management. Results are used to evaluate the effectiveness of therapy and to guide changes in diet, exercise, and medications.

1. **Self-monitoring of blood glucose.** Self-monitoring of blood glucose allows rapid and precise adjustments in treatment and monitoring/prevention of asymptomatic hypoglycemia. It also improves compliance, by allowing patients to participate in their own care, and reinforces the importance of diet and exercise. Most individuals with type 1 diabetes and pregnant females treated with insulin require self-monitoring 3 or more times a day. For persons with type 2 diabetes, the frequency of self-monitoring is based on the treatment regimen and the stability of glucose measurements; more frequent monitoring is recommended for type 2 diabetic patients who are receiving insulin or insulin secretagogues and for those not at glycemic goal. Most patients should be initially instructed to record morning and pre-dinner glucose levels. As the antidiabetic regimen is intensified and glycemic targets are approached, patients should begin checking preprandial and 2-hour postprandial glucose levels with at least one meal per day (ideally with every meal). This will allow pre- and postprandial glucose patterns to emerge over 1-2 weeks so that drug therapy can be refined. It is important to teach patients proper monitoring technique and how to adjust their diet, exercise, and medications based on blood glucose measurements. Patients should also be reminded to check their meter and strips using the control solution at least once a month or whenever they open a new bottle of strips, whichever is sooner. Proper monitoring technique should be periodically confirmed.

2. **Hemoglobin A_{1c}.** Hemoglobin is continuously glycated during the 120-day life span of the erythrocyte. Hemoglobin A_{1c} (HbA_{1c}), the major glycated subfraction, has provided a tool to monitor the 6-week to 3-month average of a patient's glucose control. (The cumulative amount of HbA_{1c} in an erythrocyte is directly proportional to the time-averaged concentration of glucose in the bloodstream and is not affected by acute changes in blood glucose or recent food intake.) Ideal HbA_{1c} levels are ≤ 5.0%, while levels > 6.0% are virtually diagnostic of diabetes. HbA_{1c} levels may be artificially low in uremia, hemoglobinopathy, pregnancy, blood transfusion, and hemolytic anemia. For patients with uremia or hemoglobinopathy, glycated serum protein, which reflects the degree of glucose binding to serum protein (mainly albumin), or fructosamine can be used as an index of glycemic control over the previous 4-8 weeks and 2-4 weeks, respectively. The American Diabetes Association recommends HbA_{1c} testing every 3 months in patients whose therapy has changed or who have not yet met treatment goals and at least twice yearly in patients with stable glycemic control meeting target goals. The assay for HbA_{1c} has not yet been standardized, and each lab reports a different reference range depending on the assay used. In the U.S., the NGSP has succeeded in standardizing approximately 95% of the laboratories, with results certified as "traceable to the DCCT A1C assay." However, the sensitivity, specificity, and accuracy of the HbA_{1c} test is still not sufficient to allow the assay to be used to diagnose diabetes, and in many countries, HbA_{1c} assays are not widely available. HbA_{1c} can also be used to confirm the accuracy of self-reported blood glucose measurements (Table 3.3).

C. **Types of Therapy.** Therapeutic lifestyle changes—medical nutritional therapy, exercise, weight control, smoking cessation—are mandatory to optimize glycemic control and reduce cardiovascular risk (Chapter 4). Five functional classes of oral pharmacologic agents are available for the treatment of type 2 diabetes: thiazolidinediones (TZD's), biguanides, alpha-glucosidase inhibitors, insulin secretagogues, and DPP-4 inhibitors (Chapter 5). In addition there are three functional classes of subcutaneous injectable agents: insulin, incretin mimetics (exenatide),

Table 3.3. Correlation Between HbA_{1c} with Mean Plasma Glucose Levels

	Mean plasma glucose	
HbA_{1c}	mg/dL	mmol/L
11	310	17.5
10	275	15.5
9	240	13.5
8	205	11.5
7	170	9.5
6	135	7.5

From: Standards of Medical Care in Diabetes. The American Diabetes Association. Diabetes Care 2007;30(suppl 1):S4-S41.

and amylin mimetics (pramlintide). Insulin therapy is usually reserved for type 2 diabetic patients with inadequate glycemic control despite lifestyle changes and oral combination therapy. Special therapeutic considerations for individuals with advanced age, acute MI, gestational diabetes, or severe/frequent hypoglycemic episodes are described in Chapter 5.

Other Therapeutic Considerations

Control of hypertension and dyslipidemia, smoking cessation, increased physical activity, weight control, and use of antiplatelet therapy, ACE inhibitors or ARBs, and statins reduce cardiovascular events in type 2 diabetes (Chapters 7-9). Treatment targets for blood pressure and lipids are shown in Table 3.2. Annual influenza vaccine is recommended for all individuals > 6 months of age, and pneumococcal vaccine is recommended for adult diabetic patients, with one-time revaccination in some (individuals previously immunized at < 65 years of age who are now > 64 years of age and who received vaccine > 5 years ago; nephrotic syndrome; chronic renal disease; or organ transplantation) (Diabetes Care 2005;28[suppl 1]:S4-S36). Screening and early treatment of atherosclerotic vascular disease, retinopathy, nephropathy, and foot ulcers are mandatory in all patients (Chapter 6). Early psychosocial assessment is recommended to identify patients at risk for medical noncompliance and depression (pp. 57-59).

Patient Education

Many diabetic individuals are unaware that they are at increased risk of heart attack and stroke and are unable to identify more than one early warning sign of these conditions. Also, more than 50% of patients discontinue hypertension, diabetes, and dyslipidemia medications without informing their physician. All persons with diabetes should be educated about the silent nature of their disease, the risks if left untreated, proper technique for self-monitoring of blood glucose, and the method for adjusting diet, activity, and medications based on blood glucose measurments. Adherence to diabetes therapy can also be improved by challenging patients to play an active role in their disease—recording blood glucose at home, reporting side effects, involving their families, challenging them to reach and maintain the therapeutic goal. Hypertensive patients should be encouraged to record and report their blood pressure prior to their morning drug dose (to ensure protection against the surge in blood pressure upon awakening) and in the early evening (to ensure coverage throughout the day). Compliance measures should be reinforced at every visit, including the importance of continuing statins and hypertension and diabetes medications.

Chapter 4

Therapeutic Lifestyle Changes

Diet modification, weight control, and increased physical activity are important therapeutic lifestyle changes for all persons with diabetes or cardiovascular disease. For patients requiring drug therapy for diabetes, hypertension or dyslipidemia, drugs should be added to, not substituted for, diet modification and other lifestyle changes.

Diet Modification

Initiation of the Therapeutic Lifestyle Changes (TLC) diet, advocated by the National Cholesterol Education Program Adult Treatment Panel III, can lower LDL cholesterol levels by 10-20% in patients previously consuming a typical Western diet (Tables 4.1, 4.2) (Circulation 2002;106:3145-3421). Table 4.3 lists other dietary measures to lower LDL cholesterol.

Table 4.1. Therapeutic Lifestyle Changes (TLC) Diet

Food Composition	Recommendation
Total fat *Saturated fat** *Polyunsaturated fat* *Monounsaturated fat*	25-35% of total calories < 7% of total calories Up to 10% of total calories Up to 20% of total calories
Carbohydrates	40-50% of total calories†
Fiber	25-40 gm/d
Protein	15-25% of total calories
Cholesterol	< 200 mg/d
Total calories	Sufficient to maintain desirable body weight

* Trans fats also raise LDL cholesterol and should be avoided

† Most as complex carbohydrates from vegetables, fruits, and whole grains

Table 4.2. Components of the TLC Diet: Recommendations from NCEP-ATP III

Component	Evidence	Recommendations
Total fat	Polyunsaturated and monounsaturated fats do not raise LDL cholesterol when substituted for carbohydrates in the diet.	It is not necessary to restrict total fat intake provided saturated fats and trans fats are minimized.
Saturated fats	High intakes of saturated fats raise LDL cholesterol and are associated with high population rates of CHD (C2). Reduction in intake of saturated fats reduces CHD risk.	A therapeutic diet to maximize LDL-lowering should contain < 7% of total calories as saturated fats.
Trans fats	Trans fats raise LDL cholesterol. Prospective studies support an association between higher intakes of trans fats and CHD. Trans fats comprise 2% of the average American diet; eliminating these fats from diet could reduce cardiovascular events up to 50%.	Intakes of trans fats should be kept low. Extra virgin olive oil, soft margarine, and trans fat-free margarine are encouraged instead of butter, stick margarine, and shortening.
Polyunsaturated fats	Linoleic acid and linolenic polyunsaturated fat reduce LDL cholesterol levels when substituted for saturated fats. Clinical trials indicate that substitution of polyunsaturated fats for saturated fats reduces risk for CHD.	Polyunsaturated fats can replace saturated fat. Most polyunsaturated fats should be derived from nuts, avocados, olive and canola oils. Intake can range up to 10% of total calories.

Table 4.2. Components of the TLC Diet: Recommendations from NCEP-ATP III (cont'd)

Component	Evidence	Recommendations
Mono-unsaturated fats	Monounsaturated fats lower LDL cholesterol relative to saturated fatty acids but do not lower HDL cholesterol or raise triglycerides. Diets rich in monounsaturated fats provided by plant sources and rich in fruits, vegetables, and whole grains and low in saturated fats decrease CHD risk.	Monounsaturated fats are one form of unsaturated fatty acid that can replace saturated fats. Intake can range up to 20% of total calories. Most monounsaturated fats should be derived from vegetable sources, including avocados, nuts, peanuts, olive oil, canola oil.
Cholesterol	High intakes of dietary cholesterol raise LDL cholesterol and the risk for CHD. Reducing intakes from high to low decreases LDL cholesterol.	Less than 200 mg per day of cholesterol should be consumed in the TLC Diet to maximize LDL cholesterol lowering.
Carbohydrates	When carbohydrate is substituted for saturated fats, LDL cholesterol falls. However, very high intakes of carbohydrate (>60% of total calories) lower HDL cholesterol and raise triglycerides and glycemic index. Diabetics are especially sensitive to excessive carbohydrate intake (particularly in the form of sugar and starches), which typically results in worsening insulin resistance.	Daily intake should be limited to ≤ 40-50% of total calories. Most carbohydrates should come from vegetables, fruits, legumes, and whole grains.

Table 4.2. Components of the TLC Diet: Recommendations from NCEP-ATP III (cont'd)

Component	Evidence	Recommendations
Protein	Substituting vegetable protein (nuts, soy foods, legumes, etc.) for animal protein has been reported to lower LDL cholesterol. Lean animal protein (nonfat dairy, whey protein, egg whites, skinless poultry, fish, etc.) improves satiety and slows gastric emptying and can thereby help improve excess body weight and hyperglycemia.	Protein intake should constitute ~ 15-25% of total calories. Plant sources of protein include legumes, dry beans, nuts, and to a lesser extent, grain products and vegetables, which are low in saturated fats/cholesterol. Animal sources of protein lower in saturated fat/cholesterol include fat-free/low-fat dairy, egg whites, fish, skinless poultry, lean meats.

Adapted from: National Cholesterol Education Program Adult Treatment Panel III Report. Circulation 2002;106:3145-3421.

Table 4.3. Dietary Options for LDL-Lowering and Cardiovascular Risk Reduction: Recommendations from NCEP-ATP III

Measure	Evidence Statement*	Comments
Increasing viscous fiber in the diet	5-10 gm/d of viscous fiber reduces LDL cholesterol levels by ~ 5%.	Dietary viscous fiber is a therapeutic option to enhance LDL-lowering.
Plant stanols/sterols	Intakes of 1.5-3 gm/d of plant stanol/sterol esters reduce LDL cholesterol by 6-15%.	Plant stanol/sterol esters are a therapeutic option to enhance LDL-lowering.
Soy protein	High intakes of soy protein can lower LDL cholesterol up to 5%, especially when it replaces animal food products.	Food sources containing soy protein are acceptable as replacements for animal food products containing animal fats.
n-3 (omega-3) polyunsaturated fatty acids	Higher intakes of n-3 fatty acids may reduce coronary events/mortality, lower triglycerides by 25-50%, and raise HDL by 8%.	Patients with diabetes or CHD should consume at least 500-1000 mg of EPA + DHA per day, either from fatty fish (2-4 times per week) or fish oil capsules (2-3 capsules per day).
Folic acid and vitamins B_6 and B_{12}	There are no randomized trials to show that dietary/vitamin lowering of homocysteine will reduce CHD risk.	ATP III endorses the Institute of Medicine RDA for dietary folate (400 mcg/d).
Antioxidants	Clinical trials have failed to show antioxidant supplements reduce CHD risk. Diets naturally high in antioxidants (fruits, vegetables, green tea, red wine) do appear to confer cardiovascular protection.	The Institute of Medicine's RDAs for dietary antioxidants are recommended (vitamin C: 75 mg and 90 mg/d for women and men; vitamin E: 15 IU/d).

Table 4.3. Dietary Options for LDL-Lowering and Cardiovascular Risk Reduction: Recommendations from NCEP-ATP III

Measure	Evidence Statement*	Comments
Low to moderate alcohol intake	Low to moderate alcohol intake in middle-aged/older adults may reduce CHD risk (C2). High intakes of alcohol produce multiple adverse effects (C1).	Alcohol should be limited to not more than 2 drinks per day for men and not more than 1 drink per day for women. A drink is defined as 5.5 oz. wine, 12 oz. beer, or 1.5 oz. 80-proof whiskey.
Dietary sodium, potassium, calcium, and magnesium	Lower sodium intake lowers blood pressure or prevents its rise. Higher dietary intakes of potassium, magnesium and calcium can reduce blood pressure.	ATP III supports JNC 7 recommendation of a sodium intake of < 2.4 gm/d sodium or 6.4 gm/d sodium chloride and adequate intakes of dietary potassium (~ 90 mmol/day), calcium, and magnesium.
Herbal or botanical dietary supplements	Trial data are not available to support the use of herbal and botanical supplements in the prevention or treatment of heart disease. Ephedrine-containing products can cause fatal cardiovascular complications and should be avoided entirely.	ATP III does not recommend use of herbal/botanical supplements to reduce CHD risk. Patients should be asked if such products are being used because of potential drug interactions.
High protein, high total fat and saturated fat weight loss regimens	These diets (like the Atkins Diet) have not been shown in controlled trials to improve cardiovascular health, and their nutrient composition is potentially atherogenic.	These regimens are not recommended for weight reduction in clinical practice.

Adapted from: National Cholesterol Education Program Adult Treatment Panel III Report. Circulation 2002;106:3145-3421.

Mediterranean-Style Diet

A. **Lyon Heart Study**. Increasing evidence suggests that a Mediterranean-style diet emphasizing consumption of monounsaturated and omega-3 fatty acids can play an important role in the prevention of atherothrombotic vascular disease. The Lyon Diet Heart Study randomized 605 patients post-MI to a Mediterranean diet providing increased levels of alpha-linolenic acid (from olive oil and canola oil) or usual dietary instruction. Patients in the Mediterranean diet group were instructed to consume more fish, fruit, and vegetables; eat less meat; and use canola-based margarine and olive oil as a fat source. After 27 months, patients on the Mediterranean diet showed a 70% reduction in all-cause mortality ($p = 0.03$). The rate of cardiovascular death and nonfatal MI was 1.32 per 100 patient years in the treated group compared to 5.55 per 100 patient years in the control group ($p = 0.001$) (Lancet 1994;343:1454-9). Risk reduction correlated with best increased omega-3 intake in the treatment group. Benefits were maintained at 4 years (Circulation 1999;99:779-85).

B. **Other Studies.** The GISSI Prevention study randomized 11,324 Italian men and women (who presumably were eating a Mediterranean diet) with MI within the preceding 3 months to omega-3 fatty acids (850 mg/d), vitamin E (300 mg/d), both, or neither. After 3.5 years, the omega-3 group had a significant 20% reduction in all-cause mortality and 45% reduction in sudden cardiac death (Lancet 1999;354:447-55). In DART, 2033 men with prior MI were randomized to receive different types of dietary advice to prevent another MI. After 2 years, the group told to increase their omega-3 intake by eating oily fish (e.g., salmon, herring, mackerel) at least twice weekly or taking a fish oil supplement daily had a 29% reduction in overall mortality ($p < 0.05$) (Lancet 1989;2:757-61). Results from the Nurses' Health Study, which examined the risk of CHD in 84,688 previously healthy women, found that higher consumption of fish and omega-3 fatty acids reduced the risk of cardiac death by up to 45% at 16 years (JAMA 2002;287:1815-1821). Omega-3 fatty acids from fish oil supplements have been shown to incorporate into atherosclerotic plaque and induce changes that enhance plaque stability (Atherosclerosis

2006;7(suppl):160,T_u-W20:3,abst; Lancet 2003;361:477-85), and adherence to a Mediterranean diet lowers levels of inflammatory/coagulation markers (C-reactive protein, WBC count, interleukin-6, homocysteine, fibrinogen) (J Am Coll Cardiol 2004;44:152-8). A meta-analysis of 276,000 individuals in 97 studies found that the addition of omega-3 fats reduced the risk of overall mortality by 23% and cardiac mortality by 32%, which was better than all other lipid therapies, including statins (Arch Int Med 2005;165:725-30). The JELIS trial involving 18,600 Japanese adults being treated with a statin for hypercholesterolemia reported that the addition of omega-3 fat (2 grams of EPA daily) decreased major adverse cardiac events by 19% (American Heart Association Meeting, November 14, 2005, Dallas, Texas). These studies suggest that omega-3 fatty acids from fish or fish oil provide cardioprotective effects that are additive to the benefits of the Mediterranean diet and statin therapy.

C. **Recommendations.** Diet modification should be recommended as part of a comprehensive program to reduce vascular risk. Suggested diets are the TLC diet or a Mediterranean-style diet (Tables 4.4, 4.5).

Table 4.4. Basic Components of a Mediterranean Diet

Component	Benefits
Omega-3–rich[1] fish ≥ 2 times per week or omega-3 supplements[2]	Reduces all-cause mortality and sudden cardiac death post-MI; lowers triglycerides (high doses) and blood pressure; anti-inflammatory effects; boosts the immune system; may help prevent arthritis, depression, Alzheimer's disease.
Monounsaturated and polyunsaturated fats (olive, flaxseed, canola oils; avocados, nuts, seeds)	Do not increase LDL cholesterol or decrease HDL cholesterol (unlike high saturated fat or high intake of refined carbohydrate). "Metabolically neutral" calorie source for people with insulin resistance. Particularly effective when substituted for high glycemic load carbohydrates.
Fresh fruit and vegetables (9-12 servings per day); use wide variety	High concentrations of vitamins, minerals, fiber, and phytochemicals[3] help prevent heart disease, stroke, Alzheimer's disease, and many types of cancer (colon, stomach, prostate, pancreatic). Minimize high glycemic load fruit (e.g., bananas) and potatoes. Choose deeply pigmented, brighter colored produce.

Table 4.4. Basic Components of a Mediterranean Diet

Component	Benefits
Vegetable protein from nuts and beans frequently	Lowers LDL cholesterol; improves digestion; may reduce CHD and certain cancers. Nuts are an excellent source of protein, monounsaturated fat, fiber, and minerals. Beans (legumes) contain high-quality protein, fiber, potassium, and folic acid.[4]
Limit saturated fats to < 10-20 grams per day	Saturated fats increase LDL cholesterol, promote atherosclerosis, and increase the risk of CHD and stroke. Saturated fats are also linked to certain cancers.
Avoid trans fats	Trans fats are manufactured from vegetable oils and are used to enhance the taste and extend the shelf-life of fast foods, French fries, packaged snacks, commercial baked goods, and most margarines. Trans fats may be more atherogenic than saturated fats. Instruct patients to avoid foods with "hydrogenated" or "partially hydrogenated" vegetable oil—these contain trans fats.
Increase dietary to fiber to 25-40 grams per day	Lowers LDL cholesterol; improves insulin resistance; reduces the risk of heart disease and diabetes; protects against colon cancer and possibly breast cancer, irritable bowel syndrome, diverticulitis, and hemorrhoids; prevents constipation.
At least one source of high-quality protein with every meal	Produces longer-lasting satiety (reduces hunger and cravings and slows absorption of high carbohydrate meals); maintains muscle mass and bone strength. Lack of protein increases the risk of breast cancer, diabetes, and osteoporosis.

1. The typical American diet consists of an unhealthy ratio (> 15:1) of omega-6:omega-3 essential fatty acids, favoring excessive production of proinflammatory, prothrombotic, and vasoconstrictive mediators of the arachidonic acid cascade (e.g., leukotrienes, thromboxane). Increasing consumption of omega-3 essential fatty acids helps regulate inflammation, thrombogenicity, arrhythmogenicity, and vascular tone.
2. Omega-3 supplements (500-1000 mg of EPA + DHA daily) should be considered for patients with documented CHD or diabetes, especially if risk factors for sudden death are present (LV dysfunction, LVH, ventricular dysrhythmias). Dose for secondary prevention is ≥ 1000 mg EPA + DHA per day (obtainable with ~ 3 gm of standard fish oil concentrate).
3. Phytonutrients are naturally occurring chemicals found in plants—many of them plant pigments—that act as free radical scavengers and protease inhibitors, among others. Examples include lycopene, beta-carotene, indoles, thiocyanates, lutein, resveratrol, ellagic acid, genistein, flavones, anthocyanidins, and allium.
4. Folic acid lowers levels of homocysteine, a by-product of methionine metabolism associated with atherosclerosis.

Table 4.5. How to Incorporate a Mediterranean Diet into Daily Living

Step	Choose	Go Easy On	Avoid
Eat omega-3 rich food at least 2 times per week	Salmon, trout, herring, water-packed tuna, sardines, mackerel, flaxseed, spinach, purslane, fish oil supplements	Raw shellfish (due to danger of infection risk, including hepatitis A and B)	Deep-fried fish, fish sticks, fish from seriously contaminated water
Switch vegetable oils	Extra-virgin cold pressed olive oil or canola oil (check the label), flaxseed oil, mayonnaise made from olive oil or canola oil	High-oleic safflower, sunflower, or soybean oil	Corn oil, safflower oil, sunflower oil, palm oil, peanut oil, other oils, mayonnaise not from olive oil/canola oil or sweet syrups
Load up on fresh fruit and vegetables	Fresh fruit: 3-5 daily. Fresh vegetables: 4-6 daily. Use a wide variety	Fruit juice (no more than 1-2 cups per day), dried fruit, canned fruit, bananas, potatoes	Vegetables or fruit prepared in heavy cream sauces or butter
Add nuts and beans frequently	Soybeans, kidney beans, lentils, navy beans, split peas, other beans, nuts of all kinds	Heavily salted or sugared nuts	Stale or rancid nuts
Limit saturated fats to 10-20 grams per day; eat at least one source of high-quality protein with every meal	Fish, lean fresh meat with fat trimmed off, chicken and turkey without skin, nonfat or lowfat dairy products (whey protein, skim milk, yogurt, low-fat cottage cheese), dark chocolate, egg whites or egg substitute, omega-3–enriched eggs	Processed lowfat meats (bologna, salami, other luncheon meats), 2% milk, "lite" cream cheese, part-skim mozzarella cheese, milk chocolate, egg yolks (3-4 per week)	Prime-grade fatty cuts of meat, goose, duck, organ meats (liver, kidneys), sausages, bacon, full-fat processed meats, hot dogs, whole milk, cream, full-fat cheeses, cream cheese, sour cream, ice cream

Table 4.5. How to Incorporate a Mediterranean Diet into Daily Living

Step	Choose	Go Easy On	Avoid
Avoid trans fats	Stanol-enriched margarine (Benecol, Take Control), natural peanut butter, almond butter	Commercial peanut butter, water crackers and other crackers that contain no fat, bagels	Fast food, French fries and other deep-fried food, chips and other packaged snacks, most commercial baked goods, most margarines
Add more fiber; aim for 20-40 grams per day	Whole grains, oats, brown rice, wild rice, barley and wheat, whole grain versions of bread, pasta, bagels	Pasta, white rice, potatoes, plain bagels, dinner rolls, egg noodles	Sweetened cereals, white bread, crackers, table sugar, honey, syrup, candy, highly processed foods, especially those with white flour/sugar
Drink at least 64 ounces of water per day	Drink 8 glasses of pure, non-chlorinated water per day. Additional drinks: skim milk (up to 3 glasses); tea, especially green tea (up to 4 cups); decaffeinated coffee	Coffee (regular), 1% or 2% milk, fruit juice, sports drinks, diet soft drinks, alcohol (no more than 1 drink daily for women or 2 drinks daily for men)	Sugared soft drinks, milkshakes, excess alcohol, artificially sweetened fruit juices

Physical Activity

A. **Overview.** Physical inactivity increases the risk of heart disease and stroke as much as cigarette smoking, yet more than 70% of adults get little or no exercise. All patients should be encouraged to obtain 30-45 minutes of aerobic activity on most days of the week. Regular exercise that increases heart rate to 60-80% of maximal peak heart rate for 30 minutes on all or most days of the week reduces the risk of MI and stroke by 50% and the risk of death post-MI by 25%. It also improves insulin resistance and type 2 diabetes (lowers HbA_{1c} by 10-20%); lowers post-prandial glucose by up to 25-50%, raises HDL cholesterol levels by up to 30%; prevents/improves hypertension, obesity, anxiety, and depression; helps smokers quit; and improves functional capacity in patients with congestive heart failure or claudication from peripheral arterial disease. Noncardiac benefits include a lower risk of cancer (colon, prostate, breast) and salutary effects on osteoporosis, arthritis, constipation, mood, insomnia, and postmenopausal symptoms. Physical activity can also delay or prevent type 2 diabetes (Chapter 2).

B. Amount of Exercise. Traditionally, exercise programs have focused exclusively on aerobic activities such as walking, running, cycling, and swimming. Recent data suggest that a strength (weight) training program is an important supplement to aerobic exercise, increasing muscle mass (which increases metabolic rate), improving insulin sensitivity, and helping maintain bone and muscular strength to prevent injuries and disability. Stretching exercises (e.g., yoga) are also beneficial. Physical activity does not need to be performed in a traditional structured exercise program to provide health benefits, and a lifestyle-based exercise program incorporating physical activity into daily living is effective at improving risk factors, weight, and long-term cardiovascular prognosis (JAMA 1999;281:327-34). This can be accomplished by encouraging patients to use the stairs, walk whenever possible, garden, play actively with children, etc. Examples of moderate physical activity from the Surgeon General's Report on Physical Activity and Health (JAMA 1996;276:522) include:

- Wash and wax a car, or wash windows or floors for 45 minutes
- Garden, dance fast (social), or rake for 30 minutes
- Walk 1¾ miles in 35 minutes (20 min/mile)
- Push a stroller 1½ miles or bicycle 5 miles in 30 minutes
- Stairwalk, shovel snow, or jump rope for 15 minutes

Exercise should not be exhausting, but it does need to be invigorating and should increase heart rate. Individuals are exercising at the right level of intensity if they can talk without gasping for breath but do not have enough breath to sing (e.g., brisk walking at a pace of 3-4 miles per hour, like walking to catch a bus). For motivated patients able and willing to take their pulse, a reasonable goal is to exercise at 60-80% of maximal heart rate (220 – age [years]). Additionally, exercise does not need to be done all at one time during the day to receive health benefits. The important factor is to accumulate at least 30 minutes of moderate physical activity all or most days of the week (which can be split in three 10-minute blocks). Health benefits may plateau at 3500 kcal per week, the equivalent of moderately intense jogging or bicycling for 1 hour per day.

C. Evaluation of the Diabetic Patient Prior to Exercise

1. **Coronary Heart Disease.** For patients initiating a moderate-to-high intensity exercise program (≥ 55% of predicted maximal heart rate), an exercise stress test should be considered for individuals at increased risk of cardiovascular disease, including:
   - Age > 35 years
   - Age > 25 years with type 2 diabetes > 10 years (or type 1 diabetes > 15 years)
   - Presence of any additional risk factor for coronary disease (e.g., strong family history, hypertension, dyslipidemia, tobacco use)
   - Presence of microvascular disease (proliferative retinopathy or nephropathy, including microalbuminuria)
   - Peripheral arterial disease
   - Autonomic neuropathy (e.g., orthostatic hypotension)

   For patients with known coronary disease, stress testing is recommended prior to initiating an exercise program to determine ischemic threshold, the likelihood for arrhythmias, and LV function at baseline and during exercise.
2. **Diabetic Retinopathy.** Patients with active proliferative diabetic retinopathy should be instructed to avoid jarring or straining activities due to the increased risk of vitreous hemorrhage and retinal detachment. The degree of diabetic retinopathy can be used to individualize the exercise program (Table 4.6).

Table 4.6. Considerations for Activity Limitation in Diabetic Retinopathy

Level of Retinopathy	Acceptable Activities	Discouraged Activities	Ocular Reevaluation
No DR	Dictated by medical status	Dictated by medical status	12 months
Mild NPDR	Dictated by medical status	Dictated by medical status	6-12 months
Moderate NPDR	Dictated by medical status	Activities that dramatically elevate BP*	4-6 months
Severe NPDR	Dictated by medical status	Activities that substantially increase systolic BP, Valsalva maneuvers, active jarring+	2-4 months (may require laser surgery)
PDR	Low-impact cardiovascular conditioning‡	Strenuous activities, Valsalva maneuvers, pounding or jarring**	1-2 months (may require laser surgery)

BP = blood pressure, DR = diabetic retinopathy, NPDR = nonproliferative diabetic retinopathy, PDR = proliferative diabetic retinopathy

* Power lifting, heavy Valsalva

\+ Boxing, heavy competitive sports

‡ Swimming, walking, low-impact aerobics, stationary cycling, endurance exercises

** Weightlifting, jogging, high-impact aerobics, racquet sports, strenuous trumpet playing

From: The American Diabetes Association. Diabetes Care 2003;26(suppl 1).

3. **Other Considerations.** Patients with significant peripheral neuropathy should limit weight bearing and repetitive exercises on feet due the increased risk of foot trauma/ulceration. Recommended physical activities for diabetic patients with loss of protective sensation include swimming, bicycling, light weight lifting, arm/chair exercises, and other non-weight-bearing exercises. Activities that should be avoided include jogging and step exercises. Prolonged walking should also be avoided. Following exercise, feet should be routinely inspected for cuts, bruises or other trauma, and appropriate foot care measures initiated (Chapter 6). For diabetic patients with

autonomic neuropathy (e.g., orthostatic hypotension), adequate hydration and avoidance of exercise in extremes of temperature are particularly important measures.

D. **Preparing for Exercise.** Well-fitting athletic shoes and polyester or polyester-cotton socks will minimize foot trauma and help keep feet dry. Prior to initiating a new exercise program, individuals with diabetes should be instructed to:
- Check blood glucose levels before and after exercising
- Carry some sort of fasting-acting sugar (e.g., glucose tablets) to treat hypoglycemic episodes
- Drink extra sugar-free liquids before, during, and after exercise
- Wear a diabetes information bracelet or necklace
- Carry a mobile phone or enough change to make a phone call in case of an emergency
- Stop exercising and notify physician if pain develops in legs or chest
- Inspect feet for cuts, blisters, callouses before and after exercise

Weight Control

A. **Overview.** An estimated 65% of U.S. adults (127 million) are overweight or obese, a number that has tripled over the last two decades. Obesity increases the risk of all-cause mortality and increases morbidity from type 2 diabetes, hypertension, dyslipidemia, CHD, stroke, gallbladder disease, osteoarthritis, sleep apnea, respiratory disease, and cancer (endometrial, breast, prostate, colon). Obesity is a powerful predictor of who will develop diabetes. Compared to women with a BMI < 25 kg/m^2, women with BMIs of 30-35 kg/m^2 and > 35 kg/m^2 have a 20-fold and 39-fold increased risk of new diabetes, respectively (N Engl J Med 2001;345:7907). Overweight adults are also more likely to have overweight children, contributing to the alarming increase of type 2 diabetes among children and young adults. Weight control improves blood pressure, triglycerides, LDL/HDL cholesterol, blood glucose, and hemoglobin A_{1c}, and it can prevent/reverse type 2 diabetes.

B. Evaluation of Overweight/Obesity. (Obesity Res 1998;6:51S-209S; Executive Summary, Arch Intern Med 1998;158:1855-67). All diabetic patients should be stratified by body mass index (BMI) to assess overweight/obesity and by waist circumference to assess abdominal fat content (Table 4.7). Increased waist circumference identifies increased risk for CHD independent of BMI and is a criterion for the metabolic syndrome (Chapter 2). (A desirable waist circumference is height in inches divided by 2.) It is also important to examine patients for features suggestive of Cushing's syndrome or hypothyroidism. Persons with suspected sleep apnea should be referred to a specialist.

C. Treatment of Overweight/Obesity. The treatment of overweight/obesity requires a combination of dietary restriction, increased physical activity, and behavior modification; patients requiring additional measures may benefit from drug therapy and weight loss surgery (refractory cases). Total caloric intake and energy expenditure (physical activity) should be adjusted to achieve and maintain a desirable body weight (BMI 21-25 kg/m^2) and waist circumference (< 102 cm in men, < 88 cm in women). A reasonable initial goal is to reduce body weight by 10% over 6 months, which typically requires calorie deficits of 300-500 kcal/d in patients with BMIs of 27-35 kg/m^2 (0.5-1 lb/week) and 500-1000 kcal/d (1-2 lb/week) in patients with BMIs ≥ 35 kg/m^2. Further weight loss can be considered once this goal is achieved. As little as 5% loss in body weight will preferentially decrease peritoneal fat and disproportionately reduce insulin resistance and improve glycemic control. Calorie deficits are best accomplished through a combination of dietary restriction and increased physical activity. It is essential to communicate encouragement, support, and understanding in order to optimize compliance. Other useful behavior modification techniques include self-monitoring, stress management, problem solving (coping with urges and cravings), contingency management (rewarding achieved goals), cognitive restructuring (changing unrealistic goals and improving self-image), and social support (positive reinforcement). Pharmacotherapy (sibutramine, orlistat) can be a useful adjunct but is unlikely to be effective long term without lifestyle modifications. Drug therapy is especially useful for patients with BMIs ≥ 30 kg/m^2 or ≥ 27 kg/m^2 in the presence of other risk factors (hypertension, dyslipidemia, type 2 diabetes, CHD, sleep apnea).

Recently, rimonabant, a cannaboid receptor 1 (CB1) antagonist, has shown great promise as a treatment for obesity. In the Rimonabant in Obesity (RIO)-Lipids Study, 1036 overweight or obese subjects were randomized to rimonabant (20 mg or 5 mg) or placebo for 1 year. Compared to placebo, rimonabant 20 mg significantly improved several risk factors, including weight (–15 lb), waist circumference (–7.1 cm), HDL cholesterol (+19%), triglycerides (–13%), LDL particle size, and CRP (–0.9 mg/L); 33% of patients taking rimonabant 20 mg lost ≥ 10% of their body weight (N Engl J Med 2005;353:2121-34). Similar results were obtained in RIO-Europe, in which 1508 overweight or obese subjects were also randomized to rimonabant 20 mg, rimonabant 5 mg, or placebo; 27% of subjects randomized to rimonabant 20 mg lost ≥ 10% of their body weight at 1 year compared to 7.3% of the placebo group. Rimonabant 20 mg also significantly improved waist circumference, HDL cholesterol, triglycerides, non-HDL cholesterol, insulin resistance, and the prevalence of the metabolic syndrome (Lancet 2005;365:1389-97). In RIO-North America, 3040 patients were randomized to rimonabant 20 mg, rimonabant 5 mg, or placebo. Among patients who completed the study, rimonabant was shown to reduce body weight and weight circumference at 1 year, and reduction in waist circumference was maintained at 2 years. In addition, in patients receiving rimonabant 20 mg/d, HDL cholesterol was increased by 24.5%, triglycerides were reduced by 10%, and prevalence of the metabolic syndrome was reduced from 34.8% to 22.5% at 2 years (JAMA 2006;295:761-75). In RIO-Diabetes, 1047 obese or overweight patients with type 2 diabetes were randomized to the same 3 treatments. For the primary endpoint, body weight decreased by 12 lb from baseline with rimonabant 20 mg; significant improvements were also observed for waist circumference (–5.2 cm), HbA_{1C} (–0.6%), HDL cholesterol (+15%), and triglycerides (–9%). The HbA_{1C} target of < 7% recommended by the American Diabetes Association was achieved at 1 year by 53% of patients on rimonabant 20 mg, compared with 27% of patients on placebo (Table 4.8) (Lancet 2006;368:1660-72). Most recently, in the Study Evaluating Rimonabant Efficacy in Drug-Naive Diabetic Patients (SERENADE), 262 type 2 diabetic patients were randomized to rimonabant 20 mg/d or placebo. At 6 months, rimonabant resulted in significant lowering of HbA_{1c} from baseline (0.8% vs. 0.3% for placebo, $p = 0.002$). In addition, rimonabant resulted in significant weight loss (–15 lbs vs. –6 lbs for placebo, $p < 0.0001$), reduction in waist circumference ($p < 0.0001$), increased HDL-C ($p < 0.0001$), and lowering of triglycerides ($p = 0.003$) (International Diabetes Federation 19th World Diabetes Congress, December 2-6, 2006, Cape Town, South Africa). Rimonabant also improved all seven dimensions of a 31-item quality-of-life questionnaire, including physical function, self-esteem, sexual life, public distress, work, sleep, and food cravings (European Society of Cardiology Congress 2004, Munich, Germany). Potential adverse effects of rimonabant include depression. If ongoing trials and long-term follow up yield similar results on both efficacy and safety, rimonabant will likely become important medical therapy for the prevention and treatment of cardiovascular disease. However, a return to baseline weight occurred when rimonabant therapy was discontinued, underlying the necessity for long-term utilization of this drug.

Gastrointestinal surgery (gastric restriction or bypass) should be reserved for motivated patients with extreme obesity (BMI ≥ 40 kg/m^2 or ≥ 35 kg/m^2 with comorbid conditions) despite nonsurgical intervention. Compared to conventional therapy, bariatric surgery for severe obesity resulted in more weight loss (1.6% increase vs. 16.1% decrease, $p < 0.001$); higher 2-year and 10-year recovery rates from diabetes, hypertriglyceridemia, low HDL cholesterol, hypertension and hyperuricemia; and lower 2- and 10-year incident rates of diabetes, hypertriglyceridemia, and hyperuricemia (N Engl J Med 2004;351:2683-93). Life-long medical monitoring and nutritional supplementation with minerals and vitamins (especially iron and vitamin D) are required following bariatric surgery.

Table 4.7. Classification of Overweight and Obesity

Category	BMI*	Waist Circumference†	Risk for Type 2 Diabetes, Hypertension, CHD
Underweight	< 18.5	N	N
Normal	18.5 - 24.9	N or ↑	N or ↑
Overweight	25.0 - 29.9	N ↑	Increased High
Obesity, class			
I	30.0 - 34.9	N ↑	High Very high
II	35.0 - 39.9	N or ↑	Very high
III	≥ 40.0	N or ↑	Extremely high

BMI = body mass index, CHD = coronary heart disease, N = not elevated

* Body mass index = weight in kilograms divided by height in meters squared (kg/m^2). Estimated BMI using nonmetric measurements = (weight in pounds x 703) divided by height in inches squared

† Increased waist circumference: men > 102 cm (> 40 inches); women > 88 cm (> 35 inches). Increased waist circumference can be a marker for increased risk even if weight is normal

Adapted from: NHLBI Guideline Report (Obesity Res 1998;6:51S-209S)

Table 4.8. 1-Year Results of the RIO-Diabetes Study

	Rimonabant 20 mg/d (n = 339)	Placebo (n = 348)	p-Value
Weight (kg)	–5.3	–1.4	< 0.001
Waist circumference (cm)	–5.2	–1.9	< 0.001
Change in HDL (mg/dL)	6.6	2.7	< 0.001
Change in triglycerides (mg/dL)	–31.2	3.6	< 0.001

From: Lancet 2006;368:1660-72.

Smoking Cessation

Tobacco use increases the risk of micro- and macrovascular complication of diabetes and is one of the most preventable causes of death worldwide. Each year, 430,000 deaths are attributable to tobacco use in the U.S. alone, more than alcohol abuse, automobile accidents, AIDS, homicide, suicide, heroin, and cocaine combined. Compared to age-matched nonsmokers, persons who smoke 1 pack of cigarettes per day are 14 times more likely to die from cancer of the lung, throat or mouth; 4 times more likely to die from cancer of the esophagus; twice as likely to suffer an MI or stroke; and twice as likely to die from heart disease or cancer of the bladder. At any age, the risk of death is doubled in smokers compared with nonsmoking age-matched controls, and the risk associated with smoking is dose dependent. Despite these statistics, many physicians do not routinely ask patients about cigarette smoking or offer counseling about smoking cessation. The increased cardiovascular risk attributable to smoking returns to baseline soon after cessation of tobacco use, emphasizing the importance of intervention. By 12-18 months, most of the increased cardiovascular risk has disappeared, and by 3-5 years, the risk of vascular events is no different than that of a nonsmoker. As a physician, there is virtually nothing more effective at improving a patient's long-term prognosis than convincing and helping him or her to stop smoking. If a physician discusses this topic even briefly with the smoker and makes a strong statement about the medical necessity of discontinuing this habit, a person's chances of permanent cessation of smoking is doubled. The use of bupropion hydrochloride (Zyban) and nicotine replacement therapy (NRT) also increases the chances of successful smoking cessation. Varenicline (Chantix), a recently released oral nicotine-receptor blocker (also a partial agonist), has been shown in one study to be significantly more effective at maintaining abstinence compared to bupropion (American Heart Association Meeting, November, 2005, Dallas, Texas). In the Studies with Rimonabant and Tobacco Use (STRATUS)-US, 787 smokers who had failed to quit on an average of 4 prior occasions were randomized to rimonabant 20 mg or placebo x 10 weeks. Subjects taking rimonabant were nearly twice as likes to quit smoking (36.2% vs. 20.6%, $p = 0.002$), and they demonstrated a 0.5 kg weight loss compared to a 2.5 kg weight gain in the placebo group (American College of Cardiology Meeting, 2004, New Orleans, LA). Recommendations from the U.S. Public

Health Service recommendations from Clinical Practice Guidelines for Treating Tobacco Use and Dependence (JAMA 2000;283:3244) are summarized in Table 4.9.

Table 4.9. Strategies to Assist Patients Willing to Quit Smoking

Step	Strategies for Implementation
Help the patient with a quit plan	• Have patient set a quit date, ideally within 2 weeks. • Have patient tell family, friends, and coworkers about quitting and request their understanding and support. • Help patient anticipate withdrawal symptoms and discuss ways to resist urges and cravings (clean the house; take a 5-minute walk; do stretching exercises; put a toothpick, cinnamon gum, or lemon drop in mouth; take several slow deep breaths; brush teeth; call a nonsmoking friend and talk). • Have patient remove tobacco products from their environment: throw out ashtrays; clean clothes, car, carpets. • Encourage patients to learn as much about how to quit smoking as possible. Useful sources for reading materials include: – American Heart Association, 7272 Greenville Avenue, Dallas, TX 75231, (800) 242-8721; www.americanheart.org – American Cancer Society, 1599 Clifton Road, NE, Atlanta, GA 30329, (800) 227-2345; www.cancer.org – National Cancer Institute, Bethesda, MD 20894, (202) 4-CANCER (422-6237); www.nci.nih.gov – *For pregnant women:* American College of Obstetricians and Gynecologists, 409 12th Street, SW, Washington, DC 20024, (202) 638-5577; www.acog.org
Provide practical counseling	• Total abstinence is essential. "Not even a single puff after you quit." • Identify what helped and hindered previous quit attempts. • Discuss challenges/triggers and how to overcome them. • Since alcohol can cause relapse, the patient should consider limiting/abstaining from alcohol while quitting. • Patients should encourage housemates to quit with them or not to smoke in their presence. • Provide a supportive clinical environment while encouraging the patient to quit: "My staff and I are available for you."

Table 4.9. Strategies to Assist Patients Willing to Quit Smoking

Step	Strategies for Implementation
Recommend approved drug therapy	• Recommend the use of first-line drug therapy (varenicline, bupropion, NRT) to all smokers trying to quit, except in special circumstances (e.g., medical contraindications, pregnant/breastfeeding women, adolescent smokers). If drug therapy is used with lighter smokers (10-15 cigarettes/day), consider reducing the dose of NRT; no dosage adjustment is necessary for sustained-release bupropion. • Some studies suggest that bupropion* may be more effective than NRT for achieving permanent cessation of tobacco use, and that some synergism between the two approaches may exist. There are insufficient data to rank-order these medications, so initial therapy must be guided by factors such as clinician familiarity with the medications, contraindications for selected patients, patient preference, previous patient experience with a specific therapy (positive or negative), and patient characteristics (e.g., history of depression, concerns about weight gain). Sustained-release bupropion hydrochloride and NRT, in particular nicotine gum, have been shown to delay but not prevent weight gain. Sustained-release bupropion hydrochloride and nortriptyline hydrochloride are particularly well-suited for patients with a history of depression. • There is evidence that combining the nicotine patch with either nicotine gum or nicotine nasal spray increases long-term abstinence rates compared to a single form of NRT, based on a meta-analysis. • The nicotine patch in particular is safe in patients with cardiovascular disease. However, the safety of these products has not been established for the immediate post-MI period or in patients with severe or unstable angina. • Long-term therapy may be helpful for smokers who report persistent withdrawal symptoms. A minority of individuals who successfully quit smoking use NRT medications (gum, nasal spray, inhaler) long term. The long-term use of these medications does not present a known health risk, and the FDA has approved the use of sustained-release bupropion hydrochloride for long-term maintenance. • Clonidine and nortriptyline may be considered when first-line medications are contraindicated or not helpful.

Adapted from: The U.S. Public Health Service Clinical Practice Guidelines for Treating Tobacco Use and Dependence (JAMA 2000;283:3244-54)

* Varenicline (Chantix), a new oral nicotine-receptor blocker, was shown in one study to be significantly more effective at maintaining abstinence compared to bupropion (American Heart Association Meeting, November, 2005, Dallas, Texas).

Psychosocial Risk Factor Reduction

Adverse lifestyle behaviors (e.g., smoking, poor diet, sedentary lifestyle), emotional factors (e.g., depression, chronic anger and anxiety), and chronic stressors (e.g., low emotional/social support, low socioeconomic status, work/marital stress, caregiving strain) increase the risk atherosclerosis progression and adverse cardiovascular events (J Am Coll Cardiol 2005;45:637-51; Lancet 2004;364:937-52). These psychosocial factors adversely affect the neurohumoral system, reduce compliance with medical therapy, and increase the risk of cardiovascular events to a similar degree as other major cardiovascular risk factors (Current Atherosclerosis Reports 2006;8:111-118). Increasing evidence indicates that multifactorial prevention efforts including behavioral/psychosocial intervention may effectively treat psychosocial distress and improve outcomes in patients with cardiovascular disease (J Am Coll Cardiol 2005; 45:637-51). It is recommended that physicians incorporate into clinical practice screening for psychosocial risk factors (Table 4.10) and use behavioral techniques to reduce psychosocial stress (Table 4.11) and promote compliance with therapy (Table 4.12). Patients with significant psychosocial distress or behavioral maladjustment should be referred to appropriate specialists.

Table 4.10. Questions to Screen for Psychosocial Risk Factors

1. How would you describe your energy level?
2. How have you been sleeping?
3. How has your mood been recently?
4. What kind of pressure have you been under at work or at home?
5. What do you do to unwind after work or at the end of the day? Do you have difficulty unwinding?
6. Who do you turn to for support?
7. Are there any personal issues that we have not covered that you would like to share?

From: J Am Coll Cardiol 2005;45:637-51.

Table 4.11. Interventions for Psychosocial Risk Factors

Type of Intervention	Targeted Condition	Intensity of Intervention
Exercise training	Psychologic distress	Less Intense: Exercise prescription plus general guidelines. More Intense: Supervised exercise
Nutritional counseling	Management of stress by overeating	Less Intense: Provide nutritional advice. More Intense: Supervised dietary instruction, weight management, behavior modification
Relaxation training	General stress and stress caused by specific situations	Less Intense: Advise patient to initiate relaxation training; provide audiotapes, videotapes, instructional scripts. More Intense: Teach muscle relaxation, imagery, autogenic training, relaxation breathing, biofeedback
Stress management	General stress and stress caused by specific situations	Less Intense: Recommend vacations, hobbies, yoga, relaxing music, pets, pleasurable activities. More Intense: Teach behavioral strategies (e.g., problem-solving, self-monitoring, appropriate goal-setting, relapse-prevention techniques)
Social support	Poor structural or functional support	Less Intense: Provide specific social suggestions (e.g., join walking groups, engage in socially altruistic activities). More Intense: Use staff as a support base, enroll patient in support group, facilitate family involvement
Health information	Specific stress situations (e.g., at work or home) or low health literacy	Less Intense: Provide situation-specific information in form of book, articles, pamphlet, audiotapes, videotapes, websites. More Intense: Discuss and answer patient questions regarding materials related to health and treatment recommendations

From: J Am Coll Cardiol 2005;45:637-51.

Table 4.12. Promoting Effective Adherence to Behavioral Suggestions

1. Use clear and effective communication; make recommendations specific and simple.
2. Schedule follow-up visits to check adherence, especially during the early practice phase, as opposed to the later, more ingrained habit phase.
3. Provide a motivating rationale for the patient's treatment regimen.
4. Reinforce oral suggestions with written ones.
5. Begin with "micro" goals for patients who are resistant to behavior change.
6. Help patients establish realistic goals and expectations.
7. Involve patients in tailoring behavioral suggestions rather than dictating change.
8. Suggest activities commensurate with patients' abilities and that provide positive feedback (factors that tend to promote a sense of pleasure).
9. Openly and candidly explore potential patient barriers to adherence (e.g., lack of personal motivation, time, family support, facilities, or knowledge; fears; job, home or other pressures; cultural issues); assist patients with problem-solving and developing strategies (e.g., self-monitoring approaches, written agreements, relapse prevention) at the time of recommendations.
10. Refer patients with poor structural or functional social support to programs or activities that will enhance adherence by providing social support.

From: J Am Coll Cardiol 2005;45:637-51.

Chapter 5
Glycemic Control in Type 2 Diabetes

Intensive Glycemic Control

A. **Rationale.** Glycemic control is fundamental to the management of type 2 diabetes. Prospective randomized clinical trials such as the United Kingdom Prospective Diabetes Study (UKPDS) have shown that intensive treatment regimens that reduced average HbA_{1c} levels to ≤ 7% (~ 1% above the upper limits of normal) resulted in sustained reductions in retinopathy, nephropathy, and neuropathy (p. 149). In addition, metformin reduced the risk of macrovascular complications and all-cause mortality in the UKPDS substudy of obese patients with diabetes in spite of only a modest (0.6%) reduction in HbA_{1c} (p. 150). Epidemiological analyses have shown a continuous relationship between glycemic control and complication rates and no lower limit of HbA_{1c} at which further lowering does not further reduce the risk of complications (i.e., lower is better). Based on these data, efforts should be made to reduce HbA_{1c} to the lowest possible level at which frequent or severe hypoglycemic episodes do not occur. HbA_{1c} levels between 6-7% are readily achieved in most persons with type 2 diabetes, especially near the time of diagnosis and when utilizing drugs that do not cause hypoglycemia (metformin, TZD's, alpha-glucosidase inhibitors, DPP-4 inhibitors, incretin mimetics). The risks and benefits of treating patients with type 2 diabetes to a HbA_{1c} < 6% are under evaluation in the Action to Control Cardiovascular Risk in Diabetes (ACCORD) trial.

B. **Disadvantages.** The major disadvantages of intensive treatment are weight gain, which is largely due to reduced calorie loss through glycosuria, and hypoglycemia. Weight gain can usually be controlled through diet modification, increased physical activity, and the use of metformin or incretin mimetics, which have been shown to attenuate the weight gain associated with improved glucose control when used as monotherapy or in combination with other agents. The risk of hypoglycemia can be reduced by frequent blood glucose monitoring; alteration of the timing, frequency, and content of meals; adjustment of insulin or insulin secretagogue dosage (if used); and change in exercise/activity patterns. The highest annual rate of hypoglycemic episodes in UKPDS was 2.3% and occurred in subjects receiving insulin. Implementation of intensive glycemic therapy also requires expanded health care teams; major professional and patient educational efforts, including comprehensive self-management training; and an enhanced partnership between specialists and primary care providers.

C. **Patient Selection.** There are few absolute contraindications to intensive glycemic therapy, although aggressive tight control should not be attempted by noncompliant patients or in patients with frequent/severe hypoglycemic episodes. Also, older individuals with advanced atherosclerosis may be vulnerable to permanent cerebral injury from severe hypoglycemia and may not be good candidates for rapid tight control, but rather a slow progressive decrease in HbA_{1c}.

General Approach to Intensive Glycemic Control

The American Diabetes Association (ADA) recommends initiating glycemic therapy for persons with preprandial plasma glucose levels > 150 mg/dL, bedtime plasma glucose levels > 180 mg/dL, pre-prandial whole blood glucose levels > 140 mg/dL, or bedtime whole blood glucose levels > 160 mg/dL. Adult nonpregnant patients should receive aggressive treatment to HbA_{1c} levels < 7%. However, the American Association of Clinical Endocrinologists (AACE)/American College of Endocrinology (ACE), and the International Diabetes Federation all recommend tighter glycemic control (HbA_{1c} < 6.5%; Table 3.2, p. 30). The Canadian Diabetes Association has recommended the goal of therapy to be a normal HbA_{1c} (< 6%) if this can be achieved without unacceptable side effects (hypoglycemia); as of 2006, the ADA has added this as an optional goal for treatment.

A. **Therapeutic Lifestyle Changes.** Diet and exercise are the cornerstones for successful management of type 2 diabetes. Caloric restriction, weight loss, and increased physical activity will improve insulin resistance, hyperglycemia, hypertension, and lipid profile. Lifestyle changes also improve the efficacy of other diabetic therapies. In some obese patients, lifestyle changes may appear to reverse diabetes. For most patients, however, once diabetes is diagnosed, at least a relative insulin deficiency is present, and pharmacologic therapy is usually required; lifestyle changes alone almost invariably fail within months. Guidelines for medical nutritional therapy, weight loss, and physical activity are described in Chapter 4.

B. **Pharmacologic Therapy.** Traditional management of hyperglycemia involved starting with a single agent, increasing that agent to the maximum recommended dose, then waiting for HbA_{1c} levels to rise before advancing/changing therapy. This passive approach has proven to be ineffective at controlling diabetes and preventing complications. Multiple classes of oral agents are now available which can be used in combination to improve glycemic control, reduce side effects, and address the fundamental defects in type 2 diabetes—insulin resistance, beta-cell secretory defect, increased glucose production by the liver, and decreased incretin production from the intestine. Combination therapy to handle most or all of these defects should be instituted early in the treatment course to achieve/maintain normoglycemia, improve insulin resistance and preserve beta-cell function, rather than initiated as a reaction to uncontrolled, symptomatic hyperglycemia.

Drug Classes Used for Glycemic Control (Tables 5.1, 5.2)

There are five functional classes of oral diabetes agents, which work primarily by: (1) augmenting insulin secretion (secretagogues); (2) decreasing hepatic glucose production (metformin); (3) improving insulin activity in the muscle, liver, and adipocyte (thiazolidinediones [TZD's]); (4) decreasing glucose absorption from the gastrointestinal tract (alpha-glucosidase inhibitors); or (5) increasing incretin levels (incretin mimetics or DPP-4 inhibitors) (Table 5.1). In addition, there is one inhaled agent, human insulin of DNA origin, and three classes of subcutaneous injectable agents: insulin, incretin mimetics (exenatide), and amylin analogs (pramlintide). This section reviews the various drug classes used for glycemic control in type 2 diabetes.

A. **Insulin Secretagogues: Stimulation of Pancreatic Beta Cells to Produce More Insulin.** Antidiabetic drugs that act by increasing insulin secretion are called secretagogues, and they can be separated into two groups: sulfonylureas and the glitinides. Sulfonylureas are one of the oldest classes of antidiabetic agents, and many are available. The two most common adverse effects associated with sulfonylureas are hypoglycemia and weight gain. Second-generation sulfonylureas (glyburide, glipizide, glimepiride) are more effective at lowering HbA_{1c} than older agents (e.g., chlorpropamide) and are associated with fewer adverse effects. Sulfonylureas, with the exception of glimepiride, abolish ischemic preconditioning of the myocardium in some patients, predisposing to larger infarcts in the setting of coronary occlusion and loss of ST segment elevation so that fibrinolytic therapy is not utilized. The glitinide secretagogues are a newer class and include two currently available products: nateglinide and repaglinide. Both products are approved for use as monotherapy or in combination with metformin. Repaglinide is also approved for use with TZD's. Compared to sulfonylureas, these agents have a shorter half-life (shorter duration of action) and a reduced risk of hypoglycemia. Because of their short half-life, glitinides are administered at meals to improve postprandial glycemic control, which may result in less weight gain and potentially less atherosclerosis and fewer cardiac events than the longer-acting sulfonylureas. In one study, despite similar improvements in HbA_{1c}, nateglinide and repaglinide reduced inflammation and atherosclerosis better than sulfonylureas, probably due to superior reductions in post-prandial glucose levels (Circulation 2004;110:214-219). The secretagogues have traditionally been employed as first-line therapy because for many years they were the only oral agents available to treat hyperglycemia. Their ability to rapidly lower blood glucose levels is valuable in the initial short-term management of hyperglycemia, but the effect is not durable (Figure 5.1) and other agents must be added to maintain normoglycemia in the majority of patients. Traditionally a secretagogue would be increased to the maximal FDA-approved dose before adding other agents to the glycemic regimen. However, data suggest that maximal augmentation of insulin secretion typically occurs using 25-50% of the maximum recommended dose, which has resulted in a trend toward use of a low-dose secretagogue in early combination therapy, and not increasing the secretagogue dose beyond half-maximum. The triple combination of a secretagogue, metformin, and a TZD is now FDA approved.

Table 5.1. Oral Glycemic Agents Used for Type 2 Diabetes

Drug Class	Antidiabetic Agents	Mechanisms of Action
Thiazolidinediones (TZD's)	Rosiglitazone (Avandia) Pioglitazone (Actos)	Increased insulin sensitivity; preservation of beta cell function
Biguanides	Metformin (Glucophage)	Decreased hepatic glucose output
Alpha-glucosidase inhibitors	Acarbose (Precose) Miglitol (Glyset)	Delayed GI absorption of carbohydrates
Insulin secretagogues *Sulfonylureas*	Chlorpropamide (Diabinese) Glipizide (Glucotrol/XL) Glyburide (DiaBeta, Micronase, Glynase) Glimepiride (Amaryl)	Increased insulin release
Glitinides	Nateglinide (Starlix) Repaglinide (Prandin)	Increased insulin release
Dipeptidyl peptidase-4 (DPP-4) inhibitors	Sitagliptin (Januvia) Vildagliptin (Galvus)	Increased GLP-1 levels; augmentation of glucose-stimulated insulin release and suppression of glucagon production; preservation of beta cell function
Combination TZD + biguanide	Rosiglitazone + metformin (Avandamet) Pioglitazone + metformin (Actoplusmet)	Increased insulin sensitivity; decreased hepatic glucose output; preservation of beta cell function
Combination sulfonylurea + biguanide	Glipizide + metformin (Metaglip) Glyburide + metformin (Glucovance)	Increased insulin secretion; decreased hepatic glucose output
Combination TZD + sulfonylurea	Rosiglitazone + glimepiride (Avandaryl) Pioglitazone + glimepiride (Duetact)	Increased insulin secretion; increased insulin sensitivity; preservation of beta cell function

Table 5.2. Antidiabetic Therapies for Type 2 Diabetes†

	Diet/Exercise	Sulfonylureas/Glitinides	Metformin
Primary mechanism	Decreased insulin resistance	Increased insulin secretion	Decreased hepatic glucose output
Typical ↓ in HbA_{1c}*	0.5-2.0	1.0-2.0	1.0-2.0
Typical starting dose	Caloric restriction to decrease weight by 1-2 kg/month; increase moderate exercise to ≥ 30 minutes daily	glyburide (1.25 mg/d) glipizide (2.5 mg/d) glimepiride (1-2 mg/d) nateglinide (60 mg)¶ repaglinide (0.5 mg)¶	500 mg bid immediately after breakfast and dinner
Maximal dose	Can use meal substitutes and add orlistat or sibutramine	glyburide (20 mg/d) glipizide (40 mg/d) glimepiride (8 mg/d) nateglinide (120 mg)¶ repaglinide (4 mg)¶	2550 mg/d (850 mg with meals or 1 gm bid plus 500 mg at noon or bedtime)
Common or severe adverse effects	Joint pain	Hypoglycemia, weight gain	GI symptoms, lactic acidosis (rare)
Advantages	No medications, improves insulin sensitivity, improves nearly all other CV risk factors	Well established, ↓ microvascular risk, nateglinide/repaglinide target postprandial glycemia and may cause less weight gain and less hypoglycemia	↓ macrovascular risk, facilitates weight loss, improves lipid profile, no hypoglycemia, ↑ fibrinolysis, ↓ CRP, improves endothelial function
Disadvantages	Poor compliance	Hypoglycemia, weight gain, hyperinsulinemia, multiple daily dosing (nateglinide/repaglinide), lack of CV benefit in outcome trials	Adverse GI effects, many contraindications, lactic acidosis (rare), anemia
Combination products	—	glyburide/metformin glipizide/metformin rosiglitazone/glimepiride pioglitazone/glimepiride	glyburide/metformin glipizide/metformin rosiglitazone/metformin pioglitazone/metformin

Table 5.2. Antidiabetic Therapies for Type 2 Diabetes[†] (cont'd)

	DPP-4 Inhibitors	TZD's	Alpha-Glucosidase Inhibitors
Primary mechanism	Increased incretin (GLP-1, GIP) levels	Increased insulin sensitivity	Delayed GI absorption of carbohydrates
Typical ↓ in HbA_{1c}*	0.6-1.0	0.5-1.9	0.5-1.0
Typical starting dose	sitagliptin (100 mg/d) vildagliptin (50 mg/d)	rosiglitazone (2 mg/d) pioglitazone (15 mg/d)	acarbose (25 mg)[‡] miglitol (25 mg)[‡]
Maximal dose	sitagliptin (200 mg/d) vildagliptin (100 mg/d)	rosiglitazone (8 mg/d) pioglitazone (45 mg/d)	acarbose (100 mg)[‡] miglitol (100 mg)[‡]
Common or severe adverse effects	None reported at this time	Edema, weight gain, anemia, long-bone fracture	Flatulence, GI discomfort
Advantages	Increases incretin (GLP-1, GIP) levels. Increases insulin release and suppresses glucagon and post-prandial glucose levels. May preserve beta-cell function and decrease hepatic glucose production. Slows gastric emptying	No hypoglycemia, glycemic durability, non-glycemic CV benefits, ↓ insulin resistance, once-daily dosing, possible beta cell preservation; ↓ in PAI_1, metalloproteinases, blood pressure, and microalbuminuria	Targets postprandial glycemia, rare hypoglycemia, nonsystemic
Disadvantages	—	Weight gain, edema, slow onset of action, potential ↑ in frequency of CHF, anemia, and long-bone fractures	More complex (3 times daily) dosing schedule, adverse GI effects, decrease dose in chronic kidney disease
Combination products	None	rosiglitazone/metformin rosiglitazone/glimepiride pioglitazone/glimepiride pioglitazone/metformin	None

Table 5.2. Antidiabetic Therapies for Type 2 Diabetes† (cont'd)

	Incretin Mimetic	Insulin§
Primary mechanism	Slowed gastric emptying, increased insulin secretion and release, suppressed glucagon production	Increased insulin levels
Typical ↓ in HbA_{1c}*	0.4-1.1	1.5-2.5
Typical starting dose	exenatide 5 mcg bid SC	Depends on insulin regimen and patient characteristics
Maximal dose	exenatide 10 mcg bid SC	None
Common/severe adverse effects	Nausea	Hypoglycemia, weight gain
Advantages	Weight loss, beta-cell rejuvenation, decreased glucagon production	Good control with intensive therapy, can be used in gestational diabetes
Disadvantages	Nausea	Hypoglycemia, multiple daily injections, weight gain
Combination products	None	Humulog Mix 75/25, Humulog Mix 50/50, Humilin Mix 70/30, Humilin Mix, 50/50, Novolog Mix 70/30

Adapted from: JAMA 2002;286:360-382. Also see Tables 5.1-5.4 and Chapter 11 for additional product information

* Drop in HbA_{1c} depends on level at time of initiation of therapy.

† In addition to the antidiabetic therapies listed above, pramlintide is an amylin mimetic indicated for patients who used mealtime insulin therapy and have failed to achieve desired glucose control. See p. 166 for pramlintide drug summary.

¶ Administer before meals

‡ Administer with meals

§ Also see pp. 160, 172-174.

B. Metformin: Reduction of Glucose Output by the Liver. The primary action of metformin, the only biguanide available in the U.S., is to reduce production of glucose by the liver and kidney. Among 753 obese diabetic subjects randomized to metformin or conventional care (diet) in UKPDS 34, metformin reduced the risk of diabetes-related complications by 32% ($p = 0.002$) and diabetes-related death by 42% ($p = 0.017$) at 10.7 years despite only 0.6% lowering of the HbA_{1c}. In addition, the rate of elevation of the HbA_{1c} was less with metformin than with a sulfonylurea (Lancet 1998;352:854-6). Metformin also reduced the progression from IGT to diabetes by 31% at 2.8 years in the Diabetes Prevention Program, with a greater decrease in younger subjects (N Engl J Med 2002;346:393-403). Because the mode of action does not increase pancreatic insulin secretion, hypoglycemic episodes usually do not occur. Metformin also has an anorexic effect, helping to curb the weight gain associated with improved glycemic control. Given these effects, metformin is typically used as a first-line agent in the management of type 2 diabetes and is desirable to have as a component of combination therapy. Metformin is usually initiated at a starting dose of 500 mg twice daily after meals and increased at two weekly intervals to a target dose of 1000 mg twice daily. Alternatively, it is reasonable to titrate metformin to 500 mg twice daily and then add a low dose of a thiazolidinedione and/or secretagogue before increasing the dose of metformin. The most common adverse events include abdominal pain, nausea, and diarrhea, especially if taken on an empty stomach. These side effects can be minimized by starting metformin at a low dose at the end of a meal and increasing the dose on a biweekly basis and/or using the extended-release formulation. Lactic acidosis is a rare but serious complication of metformin therapy, particularly in individuals with renal, hepatic, or cardiac dysfunction or advancing age. Early manifestations may be subtle (malaise), but abdominal pain, obtundation, hypotension, and tachypnea quickly ensue. Lactic acid levels usually exceed 5 mcg/mL. Lactic acidosis requires emergent and prolonged hemodialysis until lactic acid levels return to normal. Lactic acidosis is not a dose-related phenomenon, so there is no dose of metformin that can safely be administered to patients with an elevated serum creatinine. Contraindications to metformin use are listed in Table 5.3. Creatinine clearance (CrCl) should be monitored in patients receiving metformin, because at least 15% of

Table 5.3. Contraindications to Metformin Use

- Age ≥ 80 years with elevated creatinine clearance
- Renal disease or renal dysfunction (serum creatinine ≥ 1.5 mg/dL in males or ≥ 1.4 mg/dL in females or abnormal creatinine clearance [< 50-70 mL/min]).
- Congestive heart failure requiring pharmacologic treatment
- Known hypersensitivity to metformin
- Clinical or laboratory evidence of liver disease
- Acute or chronic metabolic acidosis, including DKA, with or without coma
- Metformin should be temporarily discontinued for surgical procedures and at time of or prior to radiologic studies involving IV administration of iodinated contrast materials and for 48 hours after procedure (until renal function returns to normal).
- Metformin should be promptly withheld in the presence of any condition associated with hypoxemia, dehydration, or sepsis

diabetic patients will have an abnormal CrCl despite a normal serum creatinine and no microalbuminuria. Metformin should not be started in patients ≥ 80 years unless CrCl is normal, and should not be started or continued in patients with CrCl < 50 mL/min. For a CrCl of 50-70 mL/min, metformin could be maintained in the setting of stable renal function but should be discontinued if renal function is deteriorating. Chronic use may result in anemia due to malabsorption of vitamin B_{12}.

C. **Thiazolidinediones (TZD's): Stimulation of Glucose Uptake by Muscle and Adipose Tissues.** TZD's bind to the peroxisome proliferator-activated receptor-gamma (PPAR-gamma) receptor and are unique in their ability to alter the expression of genes that modulate insulin action and lipid metabolism. TZD's decrease insulin resistance by improving insulin sensitivity in muscle, liver, and adipose tissue. They also improve surrogate markers of beta cell function and restore first-phase insulin release (the earliest beta cell change in type 2 diabetes), suggesting an important rejuvenating effect on the pancreatic beta cell, which normally deteriorates in function over time (Figure 2.4, p. 18). The net effect of TZD's is to decrease circulating hyperinsulinemia while improving glycemic control. Hypoglycemia with TZD monotherapy is rare and not severe. More frequent and severe hypoglycemia may occur when TZD's are used in combination with secretagogues or insulin but not with metformin. Preservation of beta-cell function and improvement in insulin sensitivity are the major rationales for use of TZD's as first-line therapy. These agents also exert numerous effects on the vasculature and lipid metabolism that may be particularly beneficial in patients with type 2 diabetes (Table 5.4). Rosiglitazone and pioglitazone are the only TZD's currently available in the U.S. Both agents are indicated as monotherapy in patients with type 2 diabetes or as combination therapy with a sulfonylurea, metformin, exenatide, DPP-4 inhibitors, or with insulin at lower doses. TZD's lead to more sustained glycemic control than is seen with sulfonylureas or metformin, perhaps due to their beta cell effect. In A Diabetes Outcome Progression Trial (ADOPT), 4360 treatment-naive patients with type 2 diabetes were randomized to 4 years of treatment with rosiglitazone, metformin, or glyburide. The primary outcome was time to monotherapy failure (FPG > 180 mg/dL). The cumulative incidence of monotherapy failure at 5 years was significantly less for rosiglitazone (15%) compared to either metformin (21%) or glyburide (34%), representing risk reductions of 32% and 63%, respectively ($p < 0.001$ for both comparisons) (Figure 5.1) (N Engl J Med 2006;355:2427-43). TZD's may cause weight gain and edema when administered at high doses, and combination use with insulin or a secretagogue appears to increase the incidence of fluid accumulation, which may in rare instances, due to an increase in plasma volume, progress to macular edema or heart failure if the drug is not stopped. In ADOPT, congestive heart failure was seen more often in the rosiglitazone (1.9%) and metformin (1.8%) groups than in the sulfonylurea group (0.6%). Peripheral edema usually resolves within 3-14 days of discontinuing the TZD. Weight gain and edema can be minimized by initiating therapy with low doses (rosiglitazone 2 mg, pioglitazone 15 mg) followed by slow upward titration at 3-6 month intervals. Since TZD's act on the distal tubule of the kidney to retain salt and water, spironolactone and amiloride, but not loop diuretics or thiazides, may be useful to prevent/minimize the edema. High-dose ACE inhibitors, ARBs, and fibrates may also be useful to prevent TZD-induced edema. In contrast, concomitant treatment with dihydropyridine calcium antagonists may worsen the edema. TZD's have not been studied in patients with New York Heart Association Class 3 or 4 cardiac status and at this time are not approved for use in these patients. TZD's do not have an adverse effect on myocardial structure or function but do increase plasma volume.

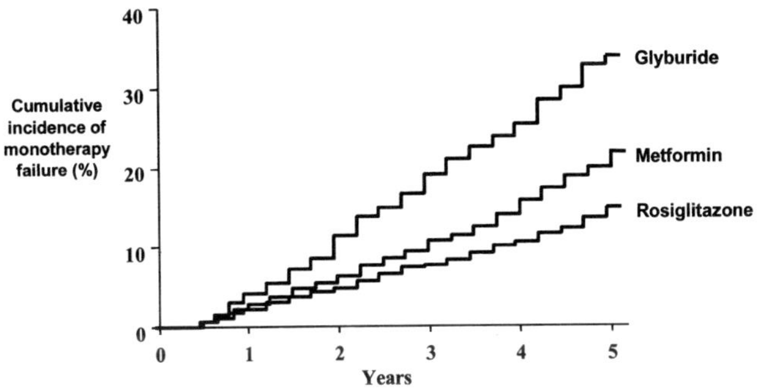

Figure 5.1. Results of ADOPT

In the ADOPT trial, 4360 recently diagnosed type 2 diabetic patients were randomized to 4 years of treatment with rosiglitazone, metformin, or glyburide. Rosiglitazone monotherapy had the most durable effect on glycemic control, reducing the risk of treatment failure (FPG > 180 mg/dL), the primary outcome of the study, by 32% compared to metformin (15% vs. 21%, $p < 0.001$) and by 63% compared to glyburide (15% vs. 34%, $p < 0.001$) (N Engl J Med 2006;355:2427-43).

TZD's are also associated with a modest drop in the hematocrit, and in ADOPT, rosiglitazone was associated with an increased rate of long-bone but not hip or vertebral fractures. Troglitazone, an older TZD, was removed from the market because of idiosyncratic hepatotoxicity. Hepatic failure is not a class effect with these agents, and rosiglitazone and pioglitazone have not been associated with liver dysfunction; routine monitoring of liver enzymes is not necessary.

Table 5.4. Metabolic and Other Effects of Oral Diabetic Agents

	TZD's	Metformin	Sulfonylureas/ Glitinides	Acarbose
Small dense LDL	↓	NC	Unknown	Unknown
LDL cholesterol	↑	↓ or NC	NC	NC
HDL cholesterol	↑ ↑	↑ or NC	NC	NC
Triglycerides	↓ or NC	↓	NC	↓
Free fatty acids‡	↓ ↓ ↓	↓ ↓	↓	↓
Insulin sensitivity	Improved	Improved or NC	NC	NC
Blood pressure	↓	NC	NC	↓
Endothelial function	Improved	+/–	Unknown	Unknown
PAI-1*	↓ ↓	↓ or NC	NC	NC
C-reactive protein†	↓ ↓	↓	NC	NC
Rate of decline of beta cell function	Improved	NC	Accelerated (ADOPT)	NC
Delay/prevent diabetes	Yes	Yes	No	Yes
Cardiovascular outcomes	Possibly improved (PROACTIVE)	Improved (UKPDS 34)	No effect (or possibly increased)	Possibly improved (STOP-NIDDM)
Adverse effects	Mild dilutional anemia, weight gain, edema, CHF, long-bone fracture	GI effects, lactic acidosis (rare)	Hypoglycemia, weight gain	Flatulence, diarrhea, liver disease in patients with renal decompensation

Glitinides = nateglinide, repaglinide; sulfonylureas = chlorpropamide, glipizide, glyburide, glimepiride; TZD's = thiazolidinediones (rosiglitazone, pioglitazone)

* Lower levels of PAI-1 are associated with enhanced fibrinolytic capacity

† Lower levels of CRP indicate less systemic inflammation; elevated levels are associated with increased cardiac risk

‡ Free fatty acids worsen insulin sensitivity and are toxic to pancreatic beta cells

↓ = decreased, ↑ = increased, NC = no change

D. **Alpha-Glucosidase Inhibitors: Reduction of Glucose Absorption by the Gut.** Acarbose and miglitol are alpha-glucosidase inhibitors that act by delaying carbohydrate absorption in the small intestine. Among patients with IGT, acarbose reduced the risk of new diabetes by 25%, new hypertension by 34%, and cardiovascular events by 49% in STOP-NIDDM (Lancet 2002;359:2072-77). Cardiac events were also reduced in studies of type 2 diabetes (JAMA 2003;290:468-94), and acarbose was shown to reduce carotid intimal-medial thickening, a marker for early atherosclerosis, by 50% (Stroke 2004;35:1073-8). Reductions in atherosclerosis and cardiovascular events are thought to be due to lowering of postprandial glucose, free fatty acids, and triglycerides. Alpha-glucosidase inhibitors are approved for use as monotherapy or combination therapy and are administered at the beginning of each main meal. The main advantage of these agents is that they are only minimally absorbed from the GI tract and are not associated with hypoglycemia or weight gain. However, they are less effective at lowering HbA_{1c} levels than other oral agents and frequently cause flatulence, which substantially reduces long-term compliance. Alpha-glucosidase inhibitors are best tolerated in patients without diarrhea at baseline. Compliance may be facilitated by initiating therapy with a half-tablet of the lowest dose followed by slow upward titration at half-tablet increments. Additionally, by limiting ingestion of starches and sucrose, flatulence can be markedly reduced, but efficacy is greatest in those who consume a high-carbohydrate diet. Efficacy can be monitored by observing a decrease in postprandial glucose excursion. Alpha-glucosidase inhibitors are contraindicated in patients with certain diseases of the gastrointestinal tract (e.g., inflammatory bowel disease, malabsorption) and should only be used in low doses in chronic renal disease and avoided if CrCl < 25 mL/min because it has not been studied in populations with low creatinine clearance, and the small amount absorbed is excreted renally.

E. **Dipeptidyl Peptidase-4 (DPP-4) Inhibitors.** Glucagon-like peptide-1 (GLP-1) and glucose-dependent insulinotropic polypeptide (GIP) are glucoregulatory *incretin hormones* released from endocrine cells in the mucosa of the small intestine in response to food. GLP-1 and GIP bind to receptors on the pancreatic beta cells, where they stimulate insulin release, suppress glucagen secretion, and reduce postprandial glucose levels. Furthermore, at least in animal studies, GLP-1 has been shown to improve pancreatic beta cell mass by increasing proliferation and decreasing apoptosis of these cells.

The incretin system is impaired in type 2 diabetes, and the decline in production in GLP-1 coincides with onset of the disease. To prevent the breakdown of GLP-1 and GIP by the enzyme DPP-4 and prolong their effects, two oral DPP-4 inhibitors, vildagliptin and sitagliptin, have recently been developed.

Like the incretin mimetics (see below), DPP-4 inhibitors stimulate insulin release, suppress glucagon secretion, and reduce postprandial glucose and triglyceride levels. Unlike incretin mimetics, DPP-4 inhibitors do not result in weight loss or nausea. Early studies suggest that DPP-4 inhibitors may improve beta cell function.

DPP-4 inhibitors are approved for use as monotherapy or in combination with sulfonylureas, TZD's, or metformin. Their use with insulin has not yet been studied.

F. **Incretin Mimetics.** Production of glucoregulatory incretins is decreased at the onset of type 2 diabetes. Since the most important incretin, GLP-1, is quickly broken down by DPP-4 when injected subcutaneously, methods to replace GLP-1 activity have been developed. Exenatide, an incretin mimetic originally isolated from the Gila monster, mimics the effects of GLP-1 on its receptor and is not broken down by DPP-4.

Exenatide lowers post-prandial glucose levels by increasing insulin release and by decreasing glucagon release and gastric emptying in response to a meal. Variable weight loss also occurs, possibly due to delayed gastric emptying, induced satiety through a direct effect on GLP-1 receptors in the hypothalamus or nausea, which is a recognized side effect. Potentially, exenatide may increase beta-cell mass by stimulating proliferation and suppressing apoptosis of these cells. To date, this has only been shown with high GLP-1 levels in animal studies; in humans, high GLP-1 levels following gastric bypass surgery have been associated with hyperinsulinemia, hypoglycemia, and at least one case of an insulinoma. In human studies, the pro-insulin to insulin ratio is decreased with exenatide, indicating improved beta-cell function.

Exenatide must be administered by subcutaneous injection twice daily. An acylated GLP-1 derivative (liraglutide), which is bound to albumin to protect it from DPP-4 degradation, is under development and can be administered once daily with similar effects to those of exenatide.

Exenatide is approved for use as add-on therapy with metformin, sulfonylureas, metformin + sulfonylureas, or TZD's. Initiating therapy at low (5-mcg) dose reduces the incidence and severity of nausea, allowing most patients to advance to and tolerate the 10-mcg dose.

G. **Amylin Analogs.** Amylin is a neurohormone co-secreted with insulin from the pancreatic beta cells in response to eating. Amylin slows gastric emptying, which can result in early satiety, decreased food intake, and weight loss. It also suppresses glucagon release in the postprandial state which, in conjunction with decreased gastric emptying, results in lower postprandial glucose levels. Amylin also suppresses hepatic glucose production. Pramlintide (Symlin) is an amylin-mimetic administered by subcutaneous injection before eating (in both type 1 and type 2 diabetes) to lower postprandial glucose levels and body weight. Common side effects include hypoglycemia, nausea, vomiting, and abdominal pain. The necessity for injections before each meal has limited the utilization of pramlintide therapy.

H. **Insulins.** Insulins can be classified according to their mode of action.

1. **Fast-acting insulins.** These analogues have a rapid onset of action and a short duration of activity so that physiological insulin levels can be achieved postprandially without untoward risk of postprandial hypoglycemia. Fast-acting insulins include lispro (Humulog), aspart (Novolog), and glulisine (Apidra). These insulins have an onset of action at 5-15 minutes, peak activity at 30-90 minutes, and a duration of action up to 5 hours.

2. **Short-acting insulin.** Regular insulin is a short-acting insulin whose use as a subcutaneous insulin has become outmoded and should now be confined to intravenous therapy. Due to its late peak and longevity of action, postprandial hyperglycemia/hypoglycemia may occur following subcutaneous administration. Regular insulins have an onset of action at 30-60 minutes, peak activity at 2-3 hours, and a duration of action up to 6 hours.

3. **Intermediate-acting insulin.** The only intermediate-acting insulin that is now available in the United States is NPH. The major disadvantage of NPH is that it is a suspension and not a solution so that multiple inversions of the vial or pen are needed—but seldom performed—before injection. As a result of this and other variables (e.g., dose and site of injection), the absorption of subcutaneous NPH is erratic, resulting in unpredictable periods of hyperglycemia and hypoglycemia. Because of this, lower doses of NPH must be utilized and targets for glycemic control are not reached. NPH is often administered once daily at bedtime in combination with oral agents or twice daily when utilized as a basal insulin in both type 1 and type 2 diabetes. NPH has an onset of action at 2-4 hours, peak activity at 4-10 hours, and duration of action up to 10-16 hours.

4. **Long-acting insulins** include glargine (Lantus) and detemir (Levemir). After subcutaneous injection, exposure of glargine's acidic solution to a neutral pH results in the formation of an insulin precipitate/depot. Detemir's longevity is due to an added fatty acid that attaches to albumin binding sites, allowing it to circulate in an inactive form until released from the albumin molecule. Both glargine and detemir have a flattened peak and a dose-dependent duration of activity up to 18-24 hours. Detemir's predictable release results in a low coefficient of variation and a lower incidence of hypoglycemia. Detemir results in less weight gain than expected, perhaps because of its attachment to albumin, its ability to cross the blood-brain barrier and influence the satiety center in the hypothalamus, or due to a lower calorie intake because of less frequent and severe hypoglycemia. Although generally administered once daily, these insulins are sometimes given twice daily in type 1 diabetes, where lower doses (per kg) are utilized.

5. **Premixed insulins** are mixtures of a short-acting (regular) insulin plus NPH insulin or a fast-acting (aspart, lispro) insulin to which protamine has been added to prolong its duration of action. These insulins are typically used in a 70/30 ratio with the longer-acting component responsible for the majority of the effect. A ratio of 50/50 (lispro or regular plus NPH) is also available.

Premixed insulins are unsuitable for use in type 1 diabetes where greater flexibility is needed. In the type 2 insulin-requiring patient, they can be used once, twice, or three times daily. Typically a once daily evening injection is given in combination with oral agents, but the HbA_{1c} target is achieved in < 50% of patients; when given as twice daily and three times daily injections, the HbA_{1c} target is achieved in 60-70% of cases. Continued use of sensitizers with these insulins can result in an even higher percentage of patients reaching goal. Due to lower postprandial glucose levels achieved with fast-acting insulin analogues, mixtures containing lispro or aspart are preferred over mixtures containing regular insulin.

Premixed insulins also have the advantage of accuracy, as mixing of insulins by the patient results in major variations in the proportion of insulins in the syringe (Arch Int Med 1991;151:2265-9.) Mixing of insulin by the patient is potentially dangerous and should be discouraged.

6. **Inhaled human insulin of DNA origin** (Exubera) has recently been approved in both the US and Europe. Exubera is in powdered form–only 20% is absorbed through the lung–and acts as rapidly as the fast-acting subcutaneous insulins (lispro, aspart, glulisine). However, studies have shown a lower fasting glucose with Exubera, suggesting that some of the remaining insulin may be slowly absorbed over time. Exubera should be administered with meals and is dispensed in milligrams; a 1-mg vial is equivalent to 3 units of injected insulin and a 3-mg vial is equivalent to 8 units of injected insulin. A major side effect of inhaled insulin is a decrease in lung function—vital capacity (VC), forced expiratory volume in one second (FEV_1), and diffusion capacity. FEV_1/VC ratios should be obtained at baseline and twice yearly thereafter. Inhaled insulin is contraindicated in smokers and ex-smokers of less than six months because of the potential for increased insulin absorption via alveolar damage. Cough, mainly after inhaling, dry mouth, and chest discomfort may also occur. Long-term pulmonary effects to date have not been assessed. Use of inhaled insulin is most appropriate for patients failing oral therapy and for those who are reluctant or refuse to use injection therapy. When used before meals in conjunction with

oral therapy, inhaled insulin can result in excellent glycemic control. However, since inhaled insulin is short acting, basal insulin will ultimately be required. Inhaled insulin can also be used as an alternative to injecting fast-acting insulins in both type 1 and type 2 diabetes.

Management of Glycemia in Type 2 Diabetes

A. **Initial Therapy.** Treatment algorithms for glycemic control in diabetes are difficult to create; ideally, therapy should be individualized for each patient. Nevertheless, algorithms are useful as an initial guide to therapy. Metformin should be considered as part of any regimen unless the person has a contraindication, given its low cost, its ability to help curb the weight gain that typically accompanies improved glycemic control, lack of hypoglycemia as an adverse effect, and its ability to reduce cardiovascular events and mortality. Both the ADA and the European Association for the Study of Diabetes recommend metformin as initial drug therapy for type 2 diabetes (Figure 5.2). The authors favor a more aggressive initial approach utilizing a combination of drugs to maximize glycemic control without causing severe or frequent hypoglycemia (Figure 5.3). Early upward titration (every 6 months with TZD's; every 2-4 months with other agents) and advancement to 3 or 4 drug oral therapy is recommended as needed to achieve glycemic control. In addition to pharmacologic therapy, all diabetic patients should receive medical nutritional therapy and instruction on exercise and self-monitoring of blood glucose. Aspirin, an ACE inhibitor or ARB, and a statin are also recommended in most diabetic patients to reduce overall cardiovascular risk (Chapters 6-9).

B. **Insulin Therapy.** When concurrent use of 3 or 4 oral agents fail to achieve adequate glycemic control, insulin therapy is required (Figure 5.4). Initially, a once-daily insulin injection should be added to the existing oral regimen. The rationale for this approach is to lower fasting blood glucose to goal with insulin and maintain glycemic control throughout the day with oral agents. To optimize postprandial glycemic control, secretagogue therapy should be maintained. For once-daily

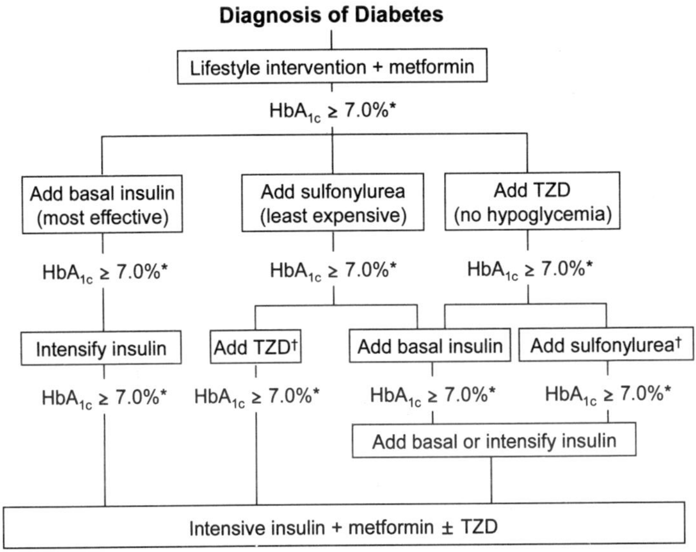

Figure 5.2. Treatment of Type 2 Diabetes: Consensus Statement from the ADA and the European Association for the Study of Diabetes

Note: This algorithm was published prior to approval of DPP-4 inhibitors. The authors favor a more aggressive approach using initial combination therapy (see Figure 5.3)

* Check HbA_{1c} every 3 months until < 7.0%, and then at least every 6 months

† Although 3 oral agents can be used, initiation/intensification of insulin is preferred based on effectiveness and expense

From: Diabetes Care 2006;29:1963-71.

insulin therapy, either premixed fixed-dose insulin containing a rapid-acting insulin (Humulog 75/25 or 50/50 or Novolog mix 70/30) can be given with the evening meal, or NPH, glargine (Lantus), or detemir (Levemir) insulin can be given at bedtime. Each of the insulins used in this situation have advantages and disadvantages (Postgraduate Medicine 2006;119:8-14).

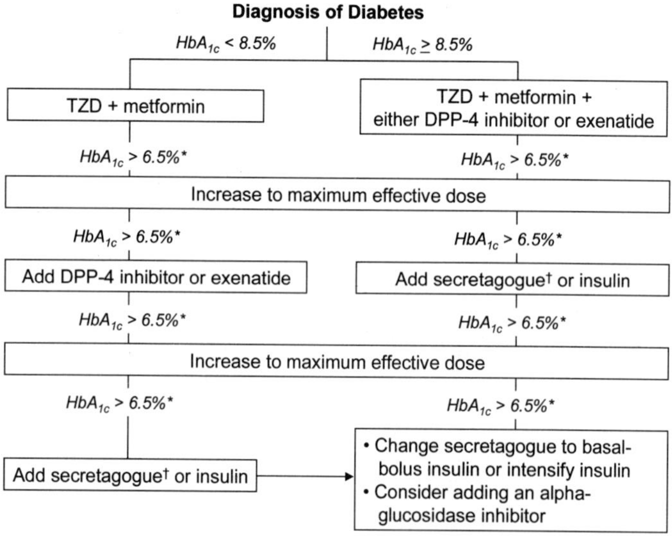

Figure 5.3. Initial Combination Therapy for Type 2 Diabetes

The authors favor a more aggressive initial approach than shown in Figure 5.2, using a combination of drugs aimed at more than one mechanism to optimize glycemic control without causing severe or frequent hypoglycemia. Lifestyle intervention should be reinforced at every visit

* For initiation/titration of TZD, check HbA_{1c} at 6 months. For all other agents, check HbA_{1c} at 3 months

† Sulfonylurea or glitinide (nateglinide, repaglinide)

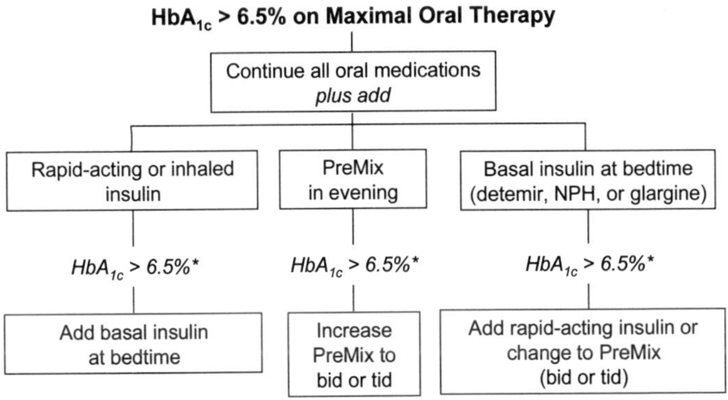

Figure 5.4. Treatment of Type 2 Diabetes with Insulin Therapy when Oral Regimens Fail

* Check HbA_{1c} every 3 months.
Adapted from: Postgrad Med 2006;19:15-20.

When the HbA_{1c} and pre/postprandial glucose targets are not being achieved with one insulin injection per day, two or more injections per day are required. At this time, a fast-acting insulin should be added and secretagogues can be discontinued. If premixed insulin has been used, therapy can advance to two injections (breakfast and dinner) or three injections per day (breakfast, lunch, and dinner). If NPH, glargine, or detemir has been used, therapy can be changed to multiple injections of premixed insulin as described above; alternatively, a fast-acting insulin (lispro, aspart, or glulisine) can be added to the current bedtime regimen and administered before one or more meals to control postprandial hyperglycemia. When three or more daily insulin injections are required, then endogenous insulin production is extremely low and the patient effectively has type 1 diabetes (near complete insulin deficiency).

Special Patient Populations with Type 2 Diabetes

A. **Elderly Patients.** Therapeutic goals in the geriatric population should be based on the patient's functional status and underlying disease processes. A healthy geriatric patient should have the same therapeutic goals as a younger patient, including normalization of HbA_{1c}. Many elderly individuals have reduced renal function; therefore, prior to initiating or continuing metformin therapy, creatinine clearance should be ascertained. Also, many elderly patients only eat one or two meals a day, which must be taken into consideration when planning therapy, and long-acting secretagogues should not be used in this population due to erratic and/or small meals. If a secretagogue is necessary, use of a short-acting agent (repaglinide, nateglinide) should be initiated once daily, which may be sufficient, and then increased as needed to 2-3 times daily, always with meals. Because of the increased risk of hypoglycemia and the increased risk of decreased intellectual function following severe hypoglycemia in the elderly, drugs that are associated with a lower risk of hypoglycemia (metformin, TZD's, DPP-4 inhibitors, alpha-glucoside inhibitors) should be favored over secretagogues and if possible over insulin therapy.

B. **Acute MI.** Optimal therapy of diabetes in the setting of acute MI consists of an intravenous insulin infusion with a goal of normoglycemia followed by subcutaneous insulin therapy once the patient has stabilized and is discharged from the intensive care unit. This strategy was shown to decrease mortality at 1 year by 29% in the DIGAMI trial (J Am Coll Cardiol 1995;26:57-65). Oral agents—metformin or a low-dose thiazolidinedione—may be added prior to discharge or at follow-up as appropriate, with or without stopping insulin therapy.

C. **Gestational Diabetes Mellitus (GDM).** GDM is any diabetes first recognized during pregnancy. A decrease in insulin sensitivity occurs in every pregnancy, starting in the first trimester and accelerating at the beginning of the third trimester. Women with inadequate beta cell reserve manifest hyperglycemia, which is associated with adverse maternal and fetal outcomes. Thus all women at risk for diabetes should be tested for

GDM in the third trimester. If diet/exercise cannot maintain preprandial and postprandial targets, then insulin therapy should be initiated. Oral hypoglycemic agents have not been approved for the treatment of GDM, though glyburide has been shown to be effective without having adverse fetal effects in a clinical trial (N Eng J Med 2000;343:1134-8). Although several oral agents have been labeled as Category B in pregnancy, metformin is the standard of care, and the use of other oral agents is not recommended. Women taking metformin at the time they become pregnant can continue the drug at least through the first trimester (and perhaps throughout pregnancy), but initiation of metformin during pregnancy has not been studied and is not recommended. While glyburide has been used during pregnancy, before or with confirmation of pregnancy, other sulfonylureas should be withdrawn and replaced with insulin. There are no data using thiazolidinediones in pregnancy so they should be discontinued prior to conception and stopped if a woman discovers she is pregnant.

D. **Severe/Frequent Hypoglycemia.** These patients require evaluation by a diabetes specialist to determine if the problem is related to insulin dosing errors or hypoglycemia unawareness. Hypoglycemia unawareness occurs as a result of recurrent hypoglycemic episodes, as hypoglycemic events that occur within 3 days of a prior episode are associated with less catecholamine production, leaving only symptoms of neuroglycopenia to warn the patient to correct the hypoglycemia. One strategy to attempt to resume the ability to sense hypoglycemia is to allow the sugars to run in the range of 200-300 mg/dL for a few weeks followed by cautious and gradual resumption of intensive glucose control. In this way, hypothalamic sensitization to hypoglycemia may be restored. Conversion to a continuous subcutaneous insulin infusion using a pump may resolve this problem. Islet cell or whole pancreas transplantation is also a consideration.

Chapter 6

Prevention and Treatment of Complications of Type 2 Diabetes

The underlying pathophysiology of both microvascular and macrovascular complications of diabetes is chronic exposure of non-insulin sensitive tissues to hyperglycemia. The presence of a large glucose flux stimulates rarely used metabolic pathways, and enzymes such as aldose reductase, hexokinase, and protein kinase C-β (PKC_{β}) are activated. As a result, substances such as sorbitol and glucosamine accumulate in the cytoplasm, which may cause osmotic swelling of cells. Furthermore, the functioning of key proteins is disrupted by irreversible glycosylation. These perturbations increase oxidative stress, which in turn leads to decreased nitric oxide levels, endothelial dysfunction, and further tissue damage. This endothelial damage to major arteries and capillaries leads to an increased frequency of macrovascular complications (coronary artery disease, cerebrovascular disease, peripheral vascular disease) and microvascular complications (retinopathy, neuropathy, nephropathy). In addition, tissues with potentially high levels of aldose reductase activity, such as the nerve and lens of the eye, can accumulate excess sorbitol, resulting in neuropathy and cataracts, respectively.

The prevention of chronic hyperglycemia in type 2 diabetes will prevent, ameliorate, or delay the complications of diabetes (Table 6.1). This chapter reviews strategies to both treat and prevent the macrovascular and microvascular complications of diabetes.

Cardiovascular Disease and Diabetes

A. **Overview.** Diabetes predisposes to a variety of circulatory disturbances—diffuse accelerated atherosclerosis, a prothrombotic state, endothelial dysfunction, autonomic neuropathy—that increase the risk of coronary artery disease (angina, acute MI, sudden death), heart failure, cerebrovascular disease (TIA, cerebral infarction), and peripheral arterial disease (claudication, gangrene, foot ulcers, leg amputation). All of these are dramatically increased in active smokers. Cardiomyopathy and orthostatic hypotension can also cause significant disability.

1. **Macrovascular disease.** Cardiovascular disease is responsible for 75% of all deaths in diabetes, and diabetic subjects without coronary disease have as high a risk of MI as nondiabetic subjects with coronary disease (Table 6.2). Diabetic subjects are at increased risk of silent myocardial ischemia and infarction, and up to one-third of diabetic patients with acute MI do not manifest chest pain. One-month mortality rates following acute MI are increased by 50% in diabetic patients, and by 5 years, cumulative mortality is 50%, twice the rate found in nondiabetic patients. Diabetes is also the most important risk factor for the development of congestive heart failure following acute MI. Following balloon angioplasty, diabetic patients have more restenosis, more repeat revascularization procedures, and reduced long-term survival. Following CABG, diabetic patients have more in-hospital deaths and strokes, more late MI and revascularization procedures, and reduced long-term survival (approximately 25% of diabetic patients die within 5 years of CABG). The risk of heart failure in persons with diabetes is increased 2-fold in men and 5-fold in women.
2. **Cerebrovascular disease.** The risk of cerebral infarction is increased 3- to 10-fold in diabetic patients, and individuals with diabetes have increased morbidity and mortality, which is proportional to the serum glucose level at the time of the stroke.
3. **Peripheral arterial disease.** Compared to nondiabetic subjects, the risk of peripheral arterial disease is increased 4-fold in diabetic men and 30-fold in diabetic women, and risk is further increased in active smokers. Peripheral arterial disease also manifests at an earlier age in persons with diabetes. In the U.S., 17% of individuals with diabetes have peripheral arterial disease, and diabetes is responsible for more than 50,000 lower extremity amputations each year. Amputation is usually caused by a foot ulcer that fails to heal and then becomes infected and develops ischemia often followed by gangrene. Since diabetic subjects often have reduced sensation in

Table 6.1. Prevention/Treatment of Diabetes-Related Complications

Complication	Screening	Prevention/Treatment
Cardiovascular disease	• Screen annually for cardiac risk factors* • Exercise stress test for high-risk individuals† • Ankle/brachial index	• Antiplatelet, ACEI or ARB, statin • Control cardiac risk factors* • Revascularization of high-grade arterial stenoses
Retinopathy	• Annual ophthalmoscopy exam through dilated pupil	• Tight control of glycemia/BP • Laser photocoagulation for nonproliferative retinopathy (severe), proliferative retinopathy, macular edema
Nephropathy	• Screen for microalbuminuria and renal function	• Tight control of glycemia/BP • ACEI and/or ARB • Possible protein restriction • Referral to nephrologist for GFR < 60 cc/min/1.73m^2
Neuropathy	• Annual foot examination	• Tight control of glycemia • Foot care instruction • Specific measures based on peripheral/autonomic neuropathy
Foot ulcers	• Self-examination for foot trauma • Annual foot examination	• Well-fitted shoes, callus debridement, proper foot/nail care • Antibiotics ± debridement for infected ulcers • Revascularization of high-grade arterial stenoses
Infections	–	• Influenza/pneumococcal vaccines • Consider hepatitis vaccinations
DKA, hyperosmolar coma, hypoglycemia (see text), screen for hepatitis		

ACEI = ACE inhibitor, ARB = angiotensin receptor blocker, BP = blood pressure, GFR = glomerular filtration rate

* Hypertension, dyslipidemia, physical inactivity, overweight/obesity, tobacco use, micro/macroalbuminuria; review family history

† Cardiac symptoms, abnormal ECG, peripheral arterial or cerebrovascular disease, sedentary lifestyle plus age > 35 prior to starting a vigorous exercise program, or 2 or more cardiac risk factors

Table 6.2. Incidence of Myocardial Infarction at 7 Years

	No Prior MI	Prior MI
Diabetes	20%	45%
No diabetes	3%	19%

their feet (loss of protective sensation) and impaired wound healing (Lancet 2005;366:1736-43), even a simple cut or callus may go undetected until the late stages of infection when amputation is required. Arterial stenoses in diabetic patients are more likely to be distal in location (tibial, peroneal arteries), making it difficult for collaterals to form and making the lesions less amenable to revascularization. (The distal location results in a lower prevalence of claudication in diabetic compared to nondiabetic patients with peripheral arterial disease.) Active use of tobacco limits patency following revascularization.

B. Treatment of Macrovascular Disease. Chapters 4-9 detail measures to reduce cardiovascular risk in type 2 diabetes, including therapeutic lifestyle changes (diet, physical activity, weight control, smoking cessation), control of hypertension and dyslipidemia, and use of aspirin, ACE inhibitors, and statins. When percutaneous revascularization is required, intensive antiplatelet therapy including a glycoprotein IIb/IIIa inhibitor is associated with improved outcomes. Increasing evidence also suggests that intensive glycemic therapy may reduce macrovascular complications (Chapter 5). Combination therapy using aspirin, a statin, an ACE inhibitor or ARB, and a beta-blocker could reduce the risk of death, MI, and stroke by 75% (Table 6.3). For patients with symptomatic claudication, cilostazol (preferred) or pentoxifylline may improve symptoms and functional capacity. For critical limb ischemia, revascularization and sometimes amputation is required.

Table 6.3. ASAB-*ASAP!* Reducing Cardiovascular Events in Type 2 Diabetes

Measure	Relative Risk Reduction
Aspirin*	~ 25%
Statin†	~ 25%
ACE inhibitor or ARB‡	~ 25%
Beta or calcium **B**locker¶	~ 25%
Cumulative relative risk reduction	~ 75%
Number of events (death, MI, stroke) prevented in 1000 diabetic patients¥	1 event prevented every 12 days

ARB = angiotensin receptor blocker, ASAP = as soon as possible. Type 2 diabetes is associated with a cluster of cardiovascular risk factors (hypertension, dyslipidemia, insulin resistance, prothrombotic state, endothelial dysfunction) that require treatment to optimize cardiovascular prognosis. Only 20% of diabetic patients meet any of the major national guidelines for control of glucose, hemoglobin A_{1c}, cholesterol, or blood pressure. Appropriate drug therapy could reduce the risk of death, MI, and stroke by 75%.

* Aspirin 81-325 mg/d. Consider adding clopidogrel (75 mg/d) to aspirin in high risk individuals or substituting it for aspirin in aspirin-intolerant patients.

† Statin (e.g., atorvastatin 10 mg/d, simvastatin 40 mg/d) to reduce LDL-C by *at least 30-40%*, regardless of baseline LDL-C. A minimum LDL-C target < 100 mg/dL is recommended. For patients with CHD or other clinical forms of atherosclerosis, it is reasonable to treat to an LDL-C , 70 mg/dL. High-dose statin ± adjunctive drug therapy may be required to reach LDL-C target.

‡ Consider ACE inhibitor in patients with hypertension, atherosclerotic vascular disease, or age ≥ 55 years with ≥ 1 other risk factor (hypertension, elevated total cholesterol, low HDL cholesterol, cigarette smoking, microalbuminuria). For patients with hypertension or proteinuria or intolerance to ACE inhibitors, an ARB can be used as an alternative.

¶ Consider beta blocker in diabetic patients with hypertension, LV dysfunction, prior MI, or high sympathetic tone (resting heart rate > 90 bpm). Carvedilol is a beta blocker with alpha-1 blockade that improves insulin resistance; beta blockers without alpha blockade may worsen insulin resistance. The addition of a low-dose thiazide diuretic (to an ARB or ACE inhibitor) followed by a beta blocker or calcium blocker may be required to achieve/maintain BP < 130/80 mmHg.

¥ Assumes annual event rate of 4%. Use of all 4 therapies in high-risk individuals would reduce annual risk to about 1%. This translates into 570,000 deaths, MIs, or strokes prevented each year among 19 million diabetic patients in the U.S. Smoking cessation, diet modification, weight control, and increased physical activity further reduce risk.

From: Freed, MS, and O'Keefe, Jr, JH. Additional references: Lancet 2002;360:2-3, BMJ 2003;326:1419-24.

Diabetic Retinopathy

A. **Overview.** Diabetes is the leading cause of blindness in adults aged 20-74 years, causing more than 15,000 new cases each year in the U.S. alone. Visual loss can occur in several ways: (1) increased capillary permeability can lead to macular edema; (2) new blood vessels that grow on the posterior surface of the vitreous in response to retinal ischemia can rupture and cause vitreous hemorrhage; (3) new blood vessels can pull on sections of the retina and cause retinal detachment; and (4) neovascularization on the iris associated with proliferative retinopathy can cause vision-threatening glaucoma. Diabetic retinopathy progresses in stages from nonproliferative (background) retinopathy to proliferative retinopathy, and both eyes are usually affected at the same time. *Nonproliferative retinopathy* is characterized by increased capillary permeability, capillary closure and dilatation, microaneurysms, scar (retinitis proliferans), arteriovenous shunts, dilated veins, hemorrhages (dot and blot), cotton-wool spots (retinal infarcts), and hard exudates due to leakage of fat and protein from permeable capillaries. Nonproliferative retinopathy does not result in loss of vision unless leakage from permeable capillaries occurs in the macular area. *Proliferative retinopathy* is characterized by new blood vessel formation, vitreous hemorrhage and retinal detachment, and is more common in patients receiving insulin. A sudden increase in the number of cotton-wool spots (microinfarcts) may signal the onset of progressive retinopathy; this complication should be suspected when impaired vision is not corrected by glasses. Retinopathy eventually affects about 85% of individuals with diabetes and is present in up to 20% of patients at the time of diagnosis. Among diabetic patients with nonproliferative retinopathy, 10%-15% will progress to proliferative retinopathy within 10 years, and half of these individuals will develop blindness within 5 years. Other eye problems associated with diabetes include cataracts and glaucoma. Blurred vision due to increased sorbitol content of the lens secondary to prolonged hyperglycemia can develop during rapid changes in blood glucose levels in the absence of retinopathy and may take several weeks to resolve after the hyperglycemia is corrected. Vision changes can also lead to insulin errors so it is important to ask patients about their vision.

B. **Treatment.** Since diabetic retinopathy is often asymptomatic until visual loss develops, and since laser photocoagulation can slow or prevent vision loss, ophthalmoscopy through a dilated pupil is recommended for all diabetic patients at the time of diagnosis and on an annual basis.
   1. **Control of glycemia and blood pressure.** Compared to conventional therapy, intensive glycemic therapy reduced the risk of microvascular complications, including retinopathy, by 25% in UKPDS. In the same study, tight blood pressure control reduced the progression of retinopathy by 34%.
   2. **Laser therapy.** Laser photocoagulation significantly reduced severe vision loss in the Early Treatment Diabetic Retinopathy Study (ETDRS) and is recommend for diabetic subjects with severe nonproliferative retinopathy, proliferative retinopathy, or macular edema. Photocoagulation destroys peripheral retinal tissue to prevent ischemia in vital retinal areas such as the macula. While visual acuity is preserved, peripheral vision, night vision and color discrimination (the functions of the peripheral retina) are compromised. Vitrectomy is indicated for vitreous hemorrhage or retinal detachment.

Diabetic Nephropathy

A. **Overview.** Diabetic nephropathy develops in 25% of patients with type 2 diabetes and is responsible for 50% of end-stage renal disease (ESRD) in the U.S. The risk of progression to ESRD is highest in Native Americans, Mexican Americans, and African Americans.
   1. **Types of diabetic nephropathy.** Two distinct forms of diabetic nephropathy exist, which may or may not be present at the same time. *Diffuse disease* is the most common form and consists of generalized mesangial thickening and widening of the glomerular basement membrane. *Nodular disease* is characterized by large accumulations of periodic acid-Schiff-positive material at the periphery of the glomerular tufts, with or without hyalinization of arterioles, fibrin caps, and glomerular occlusion.
   2. **Progression of Diabetic Nephropathy.** Regardless of form, diabetic

nephropathy may be "silent" for 10-15 years and commonly progresses in stages:

a. **Hyperfiltration of kidneys.** Hyperglycemia leads to an increase in renal blood flow, hyperfiltration, and increased glomerular pressure. Because of this, the glomerular filtration rate (GFR) may be 40% or more above normal in the early stages of the disease.
b. **Appearance of microalbuminuria.** Microalbuminuria is defined as urinary albumin excretion 30-299 mg/24 h (or 30-299 mcg/mg creatinine on a spot collection). Microalbuminuria, as well as being the earliest warning sign for diabetic nephropathy, is also associated with increased cardiovascular mortality and is an indication for screening for atherosclerotic vascular disease and aggressive risk factor modification. Microalbuminuria can be a marker of generalized endothelial dysfunction since the glomerulus is an arteriole and therefore can act as a "window" to the vasculature. All persons with type 2 diabetes should be tested for microalbuminuria at the time of diagnosis and annually thereafter by an albumin-to-creatinine ratio in a spot urine. Positive tests with reagent-tablets or dipstick should be confirmed using another test.
c. **Onset of macroalbuminuria** (urinary albumin excretion ≥ 300 mg/24 h or ≥ 300 mcg/mg creatinine on a spot collection).
d. **Decline in GFR.** Once macroalbuminuria begins, renal function untreated typically declines at a rate of approximately 1 cc/min/month. Azotemia usually begins 2-3 years after macroalbuminuria is detected. Deterioration in renal function is accelerated by concomitant hypertension.
e. **Progression to end-stage renal disease.** This has typically been more common in type 1 diabetes than in type 2 diabetes.

B. **Treatment.** Interventions to slow the progression of diabetic nephropathy include: tight glycemic and blood pressure control; an ACE inhibitor and/or an ARB for type 2 diabetic patients with hypertension and/or microalbuminuria; an ACE inhibitor and/or an ARB for type 2 diabetic patients with hypertension, macroalbuminuria, and renal insufficiency (creatinine > 1.5 mg/dL); and possibly protein restriction

(≤ 0.8 gm/kg body weight/day) with the onset of overt nephropathy. Patients receiving ACE inhibitors or ARBs should be monitored for hyperkalemia and azotemia, and these agents are contraindicated during the prepregnancy period and during pregnancy (Chapter 7). The goal of therapy, particularly in the setting of microalbuminuria, is to reduce urine albumin levels to the normal range. Nondihydropyridine calcium antagonists and/or beta-blockers can be used for patients intolerant to ACE inhibitors/ARBs. Referral to a nephrologist is recommended for patients with GFR < 60 cc/min/1.73m^2. Patients should be instructed to promptly report symptoms of urinary tract infection (dysuria, frequency, hematuria, fever, chills, flank or lower abdominal pain/pressure).

Diabetic Neuropathy

Persons with type 2 diabetes are at increased risk of developing peripheral and autonomic neuropathies. *Peripheral polyneuropathy* is associated with sensory symptoms such as numbness, pain, and hyperesthesias. Most patients with diabetic neuropathic pain will require drug therapy (e.g., tramadol, pregabalin [Lycica], duloxetine [Cymbalta], amitriptyline, capsaicin cream). *Mononeuropathy* can also occur and manifests as sudden onset of wrist drop, foot drop, or cranial nerve paralysis (III, IV, VI, VII). Spontaneous remission almost always occurs over a 6-12 week period due to revascularization of the nerve. Infrequently, *radiculopathy* can develop, and when it involves one or more dermatomes in the chest wall or abdomen, it can mimic acute myocardial infarction, herpes zoster, or acute abdomen. Radiculopathy almost invariably resolves. *Autonomic neuropathy* can affect many organs and result in a variety of abnormalities, including esophageal dysmotility, bladder dysfunction/paralysis, erectile dysfunction, gastroparesis with delayed gastric emptying and early satiety, small bowel dysfunction (diabetic diarrhea), Charcot's joint (dislocation/collapse of one or more joints or bones in foot), abnormal sweat production (anhidrosis or hyperhidrosis), and cardiac dysfunction (orthostatic hypotension, tachycardia). Tight glucose control can slow/prevent the development of diabetic neuropathy. Patients with peripheral neuropathy should take special precautions during exercise (Chapter 4) and require special attention to foot care. *Entrapment neuropathies* such as carpal tunnel syndrome, ulnar entrapment at the elbow, meralgia paresthetica, and foot drop due to common peroneal palsy are more common with diabetes. Reasons for this include excess collagen production (from protein glycosylation) and increased vulnerability of the diabetic nerve to external pressure.

Diabetic Foot Ulcers

Due to "clawing" of the neuropathic foot, which is caused by weakness of the interossei and excess pressure on the metatarsal heads accompanying a loss of protective sensation, ulceration of the plantar surface of the foot may occur (Lancet 2005;366:1736-43). The frequent coexistence of peripheral arterial disease and impaired wound healing contribute to the development and progression of ulcers, which are frequently complicated by polymicrobial infection. Measures to reduce the development and progression of foot ulcers include the use of well-fitting walking shoes, callus debridement, revascularization for significant peripheral arterial disease (J Am Coll Cardiol 2006;47:921-9), and patient education about the need for daily foot monitoring, proper foot and nail care, and selection of appropriate footwear. Treatment of foot ulcers requires adequate antimicrobial therapy, debridement, and complete absence of weight bearing so that the ulcer can heal from the base. To achieve healing and avoid weight bearing, contact casting or a protective boot may be needed since most patients are not compliant with bed rest. When an ulcer is failing to heal, vascular insufficiency or underlying osteomyelitis should be considered and treated appropriately. Unfortunately, the diagnosis of osteomyelitis may require a bone biopsy because changes in x-rays/bone scan caused by increased blood flow secondary to arteriovenous shunting from autonomic neuropathy can mimic osteomyelitis.

Infection

Urinary tract and skin infections are especially common and more severe in diabetic patients, possibly due to impaired leukocyte function. Patients with diabetes are also predisposed to several types of unusual infections. *Rhinocerebral mucormycosis* is a fungal infection that usually develops during or after an episode of diabetic ketoacidosis. Manifestations include sudden periorbital swelling with bloody nasal discharge and black, necrotic nasal mucosa. Cranial nerve palsies and cavernous sinus thrombosis can occur. This condition may present as failure to wake from coma upon treatment of diabetic ketoacidosis. Treatment consists of antifungal therapy and emergency surgical debridement. Without prompt intervention, death usually occurs within 2 weeks. *Malignant external otitis* presents with severe ear pain, fever, leukocytosis, and ear drainage and is often caused by Pseudomonas aeruginosa infecting a relatively ischemic "watershed" area of the external auditory canal. Cranial nerve palsies can occur, and facial nerve involvement is associated with a 50% mortality rate. Treatment consists of urgent debridement plus broad-spectrum antibiotics. *Emphysematous cholecystitis* presents with right upper quadrant pain, fever, and gas in the gallbladder wall on flat plate of the abdomen. Clostridium and other gas-producing organisms are frequently present, and this condition is associated with a higher incidence of gallbladder gangrene and perforation than typical cholecystitis. *Emphysematous pyelonephritis* is diagnosed by gas in the kidney or perirenal space in a patient with pyelonephritis. Antibiotics are often ineffective, and surgical drainage or nephrectomy may be required. Mortality rates may be as high as 80%. *Necrotizing fasciitis* is an infection that rapidly spreads through the tissue planes of the abdominal wall and is usually secondary to a trivial infection. Treatment consists of urgent antimicrobial therapy and surgical debridement of necrotic tissue. Mortality rates are very high.

Diabetic Ketoacidosis

Diabetic ketoacidosis (DKA) is a medical emergency that can progress rapidly to coma and death without prompt hospitalization and treatment. DKA develops when, with very low insulin levels, the body is unable to metabolize glucose and instead breaks down fat for energy, resulting in the accumulation of ketones in the blood. DKA is much more common in type 1 diabetes, where it can occur spontaneously and may be the initial manifestation of diabetes, but it can also develop in people with type 2 diabetes following acute physical stress (infection, surgery, myocardial infarction), emotional stress, prolonged hyperglycemia, or after discontinuation of insulin therapy. Symptoms usually consist of excessive urination and thirst, nausea, vomiting, and abdominal pain due to ketosis. Affected individuals often present with very rapid and shallow breathing due to acidosis and have a fruity smell to their breath (like nail polish remover). An anion gap metabolic acidosis is present and often severe. DKA is treated with intravenous insulin, fluids and electrolytes, gradual reduction of blood sugar, occasional small doses of bicarbonate for severe acidosis, and treatment of intercurrent illness (e.g., infection, MI). There are many possible protocols; one is shown in Table 6.4. All patients with unexplained DKA and type 2 diabetes should have an ECG and troponin levels checked immediately to exclude an MI.

Hyperosmolar Coma

This serious complication usually develops in elderly type 2 diabetic patients following an acute illness (e.g., infection, stroke) or following institution of peritoneal dialysis or diuretic therapy. Hyperosmolar coma may be the initial presentation of type 2 diabetes. The predominant pathophysiology is severe dehydration so that the kidney cannot excrete glucose, resulting in serum glucose levels that often reach extreme levels (> 1000 mg/dL). The most common symptom is increasing lethargy, which can progress to loss of consciousness over a period of days. Treatment consists of intravenous fluids and electrolytes, gradual reduction of blood glucose levels, and treatment of intercurrent illness. The prognosis is far worse than for DKA, and the vast majority of patients who recover do not need insulin to control their diabetes.

Hypoglycemia

Hypoglycemia usually occur in diabetic subjects who have taken too much insulin or insulin secretagogues. Severe hypoglycemia is extremely rare with metformin, thiazolidinediones, DPP-4 inhibitors, or alpha-glucosidase inhibitors when not used in combination with insulin or sulfonylureas. Symptoms include sweating, tremor, palpitations, and weakness. At lower blood glucose levels, neuroglycopenia occurs and can present as irritability, confusion, double vision, slurred speech, or coma. If hypoglycemia is prolonged/severe, seizures, accidental injury, and irreversible brain damage can occur. Hypoglycemic episodes are treated by sugar-containing foods, intravenous glucose, or glucagon to raise blood sugar levels. Special therapeutic considerations for patients with frequent/severe hypoglycemia are described in Chapter 5.

Other Complications of Diabetes

Persons with diabetes are predisposed to *fatty infiltration of the liver* and to a variety of *skin disorders*, including necrobiosis lipoidica diabeticorum (plaque with central yellowish area and brownish border over the anterior legs with or without ulceration); diabetic dermopathy (small rounded raised plaques over the anterior tibial surface); bullous diabeticorum (uncommon; bullae may be hemorrhagic or clear); skin infections with Candida and dermatophytes; bacterial infections; vaginal moniliasis; atrophy of adipose tissue (at site of insulin injections), which is rare with human insulin; hypertrophy of fat; scleredema (common benign thickening of skin over shoulders and upper back); Dupuytren's contractions of joints; and frozen shoulder.

Table 6.4. Guidelines for Management of Diabetic Ketoacidosis

Establish diagnosis

- Measure serum glucose and ketones and arterial blood gas
- Obtain complete blood cell count, serum electrolytes, renal profile (BUN, creatinine)
- Obtain fresh-voided urine sample for urinalysis
- Record pulse, blood pressure (lying/sitting, if possible), respiratory rate, temperature
- Eliminate other causes of acidosis (uremia, alcoholism, salicylate overdose)

If ketoacidosis is confirmed¶

- Admit to diabetes unit
- Discontinue all food orally
- Give 10 U regular insulin intravenously immediately
- Start normal saline infusion at 500 mL/hr IV for first 2 hours then 200 mL/hr*
- Add 100 U regular insulin to 500 mL saline solution. Dispose of first 50 mL through tubing. Piggyback to IV line and infuse at 0.5 mL/kg/hr
- Obtain electrocardiogram and institute cardiac monitoring when appropriate
- Measure serum potassium level; if < 5.5 mEq/L and there is reasonable urine output, add potassium chloride 20 mEq/L

Monitor hourly to:

- Adjust insulin. Infuse 5 mL/hr to maintain decrease in serum glucose at 50-150 mg/dL per hour and to keep serum glucose > 250 mg/dL until hydration improves
- Record vital signs and determine fluid input/output†
- Measure glucose level
- Test all urine for ketones (hourly if catheter is in situ)‡

Monitor every 2 hours for serum glucose, electrolytes, renal profile

Monitor every 6 hours for serum magnesium and serum phosphate

When serum glucose falls below 250 mg/dL

- Change IV to 5% dextrose in normal saline solution and run at 150 mL/hr. Reduce insulin infusion by 50%

When serum glucose is below 250 mg/dL, serum and urine are free of ketones, and electrolytes are normal

- Start an ADA diet and administer short-or fast-acting insulin subcutaneously before meals and NPH or glargine insulin at bedtime. Discontinue IV fluids and IV insulin 1-2 hours after first insulin injection. Continue to monitor glucose every 2 hours

¶ Correct precipitating event, if present (e.g., infection, GI bleed, PE, MI). Be aware of severe/uncommon complications (DVT, PE, MI, ARDS, cerebral edema, infection, etc.)

* Patients with severe hypotension/hypovolemia may require higher infusion rates. Monitor for signs of heart failure in patients with LV dysfunction.

† An indwelling urinary catheter is seldom needed and increases the risk of infection.

‡ The level of measured ketones may increase during clinical improvement. This is due to a shift from beta-hydroxybutyrate production to the less acidic acetoacetate or acetone bodies, giving the false impression that the ketotic state is getting worse.

Chapter 7

Control of Dyslipidemia in Type 2 Diabetes

Overview of Diabetic Dyslipidemia

A. **Introduction.** Elevated plasma levels of total cholesterol and LDL cholesterol (LDL-C) and low plasma levels of HDL cholesterol (HDL-C) are major modifiable lipid risk factors for atherothrombotic vascular disease. It has been estimated that for each 1% decrease in LDL-C and each 1% increase in HDL-C, the risk for cardiovascular events falls by 2% and 3%, respectively. Dramatic results from the Collaborative Atorvastatin Diabetes Study (CARDS) and the Heart Protection Study (HPS) have shown that statins reduce major cardiovascular events by 25-37% and stroke by 13-48% in patients with type 2 diabetes, including subjects with "normal" LDL-C levels (Tables 7.1, 7.2). Optimization of the lipid profile is the *single most important intervention* for improving cardiovascular prognosis in type 2 diabetes, reducing the risk of coronary death, MI, stroke, and revascularization procedures. In Steno-2, 70% of the 47% reduction in cardiovascular risk attributable to intensive multifactorial intervention was due to improvements in lipid profile (N Engl J Med 2003;348:383-93).

B. **Lipid Profile.** Diabetic dyslipidemia is characterized by elevated triglycerides (≥ 150 mg/dL), depressed HDL-C (< 40 mg/dL), and elevated small dense LDL-C particles, which are easily oxidized and highly atherogenic. LDL-C levels are generally normal to moderately elevated and no different than levels in nondiabetic patients. Patients with diabetic dyslipidemia often have rapid progression of CHD due to highly atherogenic LDL-C particles, prothrombogenic hemostatic function (impaired fibrinolysis, activated platelets and Factor VIII), and endothelial dysfunction. It has been estimated that diabetic dyslipidemia confers a cardiovascular risk similar to an LDL-C level of 150-220 mg/dL (Circulation 1997;95:1-4).

C. **Lipid Therapy and the New CHD Paradigm.** It has now been established that the most dangerous (i.e., rupture-prone) atherosclerotic plaques are not necessarily those causing the most severe narrowing, and that most acute coronary syndromes are caused by lesions that were less than 70% stenotic (nonobstructive) prior to ulceration and thrombosis. Nonobstructive plaques with extensive inflammation (stimulated by oxidized lipoproteins in the vessel wall), lipid-rich cores, and thin fibrous caps are more prone to ulceration and rupture than long-standing obstructive lesions with extensive calcification and thick fibrous caps comprised of dense collagenous tissue.

Moderate reductions in LDL-C slow the progression of coronary disease in most patients, and lesion regression is more frequent with LDL-C reduction. Nevertheless, the beneficial effects of lipid therapy are due more to plaque stabilization than to changes in stenosis severity, which are generally modest and disproportionate to the 25-50% reduction in major cardiovascular events. Plaque stabilization, which can be accomplished in weeks to months with aggressive treatment of dyslipidemia, may be related to resorption of macrophage and extracellular lipid deposits, a decrease in neointimal inflammation, and maintenance of fibrous cap integrity. Effective treatment transforms the inflamed, friable plaque into a stable, fibrotic plaque that is less prone to ulceration, rupture, and thrombosis. In addition, lipid-modifying drug therapy improves endothelial dysfunction caused by dyslipidemia, resulting in additional vasodilatory, antithrombotic, and anti-inflammatory effects. Treatment of dyslipidemia and other concomitant risk factors is essential to improving long-term cardiovascular prognosis in type 2 diabetes.

Intensive LDL Lowering and Cardiovascular Prognosis: Lower is Better

A. **Overview.** Recent, large-scale, randomized trials have demonstrated improved cardiovascular prognosis through intensive LDL-C lowering, prompting the National Cholesterol Education Program (NCEP) Adult Treatment Panel (ATP) III and the American Heart Association

(AHA)/American College of Cardiology (ACC) to issue guideline updates recommending expanded and more intensive use of lipid-modifying drug therapy, particularly statins (Circulation 2004;110:227-239, Circulation 2006;113:2363-2372). Data from epidemiological studies and clinical trials have shown that for every 1 mg/dL reduction in LDL, the relative risk for CHD is reduced by 1% (Figure 7.1). Benefits extend to LDL-C levels of 50-70 mg/dL, well below the previously recommended LDL-C target of < 100 mg/dL for high-risk patients. Average cholesterol levels in the U.S. are nearly twice the normal physiological level (Figure 7.2).

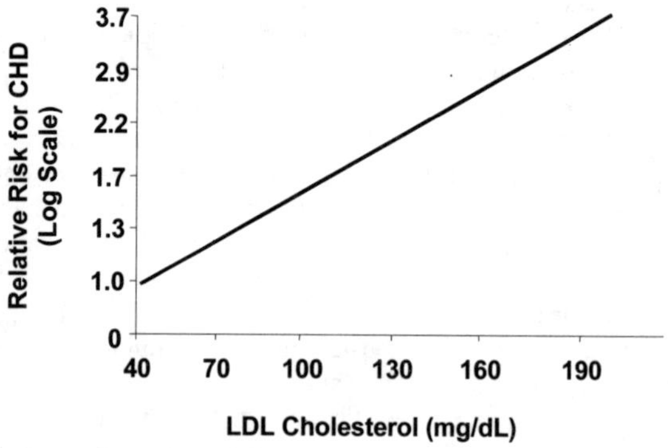

Figure 7.1. Relationship Between LDL Cholesterol Levels and Relative Risk for CHD

The log-linear relationship between LDL-C and CHD risk is consistent with a large body of data from epidemiological studies and clinical trials. For every 30 mg/dL change in LDL-C, the relative risk for CHD is changed in proportion by about 30%. The relative risk is set at 1.0 for LDL-C = 40 mg/dL. From: NCEP ATP III guideline update (Circulation 2004;110:227-239).

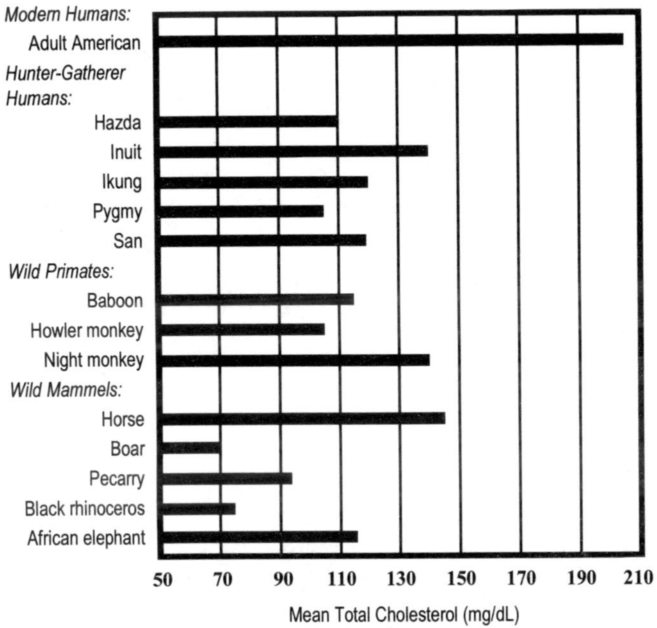

Figure 7.2. Total Cholesterol Levels in Various Populations

Total cholesterol levels for hunter-gatherers, wild primates, and wild mammals generally range from 70-140 mg/dL (LDL-C 35-70 mg/dL). In modern Westernized humans, mean total cholesterol levels (208 mg/dL; LDL-C 130 mg/dL) are almost twice these normal values, and atherosclerosis is present in up to 50% of individuals by age 50 (Arterioscler Thromb Vasc Biol 2002;22:849-54). In contrast, evidence from hunter-gatherer populations following the indigenous homosapien lifestyle indicate average total cholesterol levels of 100-150 mg/dL (LDL-C 50-75 mg/dL) and no evidence for atherosclerosis, even in individuals living into the eighth decade of life (Eur J Clin Nutr 2002;56:S42-52).

B. Dyslipidemia Trials in the General Population

1. **Placebo-Controlled Trials.** A meta-analysis of more than 30 trials using diet, drugs, or surgery to lower cholesterol has shown that for every 1% total cholesterol is lowered, total mortality is reduced by 1.1% (Circulation 1995;91:2274-82; Circulation 1998;97:946-52). Statins are overwhelmingly the drug class of choice for improving dyslipidemia and cardiovascular prognosis. In addition to lowering LDL-C levels by 18-55%, they also reduce the number of small, dense (atherogenic) LDL-C particles, raise HDL-C levels by 5-15%, and lower triglycerides by 7-30%. When CHD event rates are plotted against LDL-C levels, a direct relationship is apparent, without a lower threshold, in both primary and secondary prevention trials (Figures 7.3, 7.4). In the Heart Protection Study (HPS), the largest statin study to date, 20,536 patients with arterial occlusive disease or diabetes were randomized to simvastatin 40 mg/d or placebo. At 5 years, simvastatin reduced the risk of coronary death by 18% (5.7% vs. 6.9%, $p = 0.0005$) (Lancet 2002;360:7-22). Patients with baseline LDL-C < 100 mg/dL (~ 70 mg/dL or less on treatment) had the same relative risk reduction as patients with baseline LDL-C > 100 mg/dL. In the Anglo-Scandinavian Cardiac Outcomes Trial (ASCOT) (Lancet 2003;361:1149) and the Collaborative Atorvastatin Diabetes Study (CARDS) (Lancet 2004;364:685-96), statins reduced the risk of CHD by 25-37% compared to placebo, with benefits extending to patients with baseline LDL-C < 116 mg/dL (~ 80 mg/dL or less on treatment). In these studies, statin therapy was well tolerated and extremely safe: muscle and liver side effects were similar to placebo and rhabdomyolysis was very rare.
2. **Statin vs. Statin Trials.** The most direct evidence to support the "lower-is-better" hypothesis comes from the Pravastatin or Atorvastatin Evaluation and Infection Trial (PROVE IT), the Treating to New Targets (TNT) trial, and the Incremental Decrease in Endpoints through Aggressive Lipid lowering (IDEAL) trial.
   a. **PROVE IT.** This trial randomized 4162 patients with an acute coronary syndrome to in-hospital initiation of intensive LDL-C lowering with atorvastatin 80 mg/d (median LDL-C 62 mg/dL) or standard LDL-C lowering with pravastatin 40 mg/d (median LDL-C 95 mg/dL). At 2 years, atorvastatin reduced the primary endpoint of death, MI, unstable angina requiring hospitalization, revascularization after 30 days, and stroke by 16% (22.4% vs.

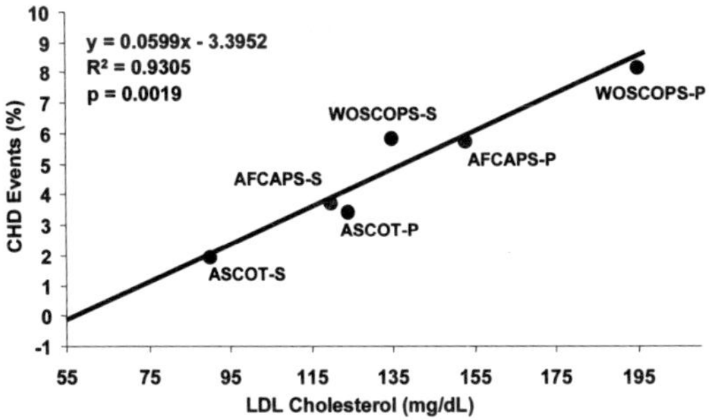

Figure 7.3. Relationship Between LDL Cholesterol and CHD Event Rates in Primary Prevention Trials

CHD event rates in primary prevention trials (4-5 years' duration) are directly proportional to LDL-C levels. P = placebo, S = statin. From: J Am Coll Cardiol 2004;43:2142-6.

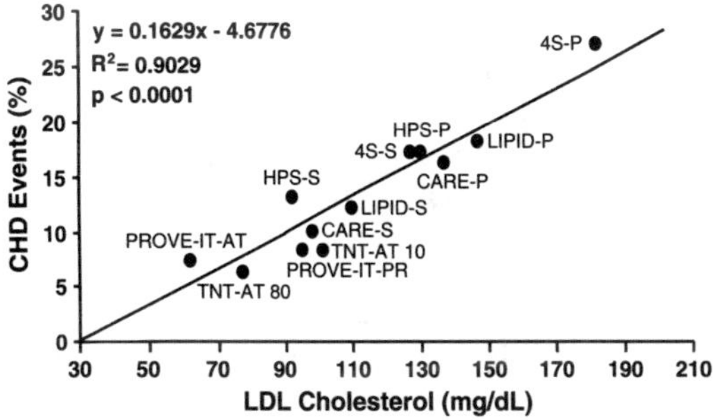

Figure 7.4. Relationship Between LDL Cholesterol and CHD Event Rates in Secondary Prevention Trials

CHD event rates in secondary prevention trials (5 years' duration except PROVE IT [2 years]) are directly proportional to LDL-C levels. AT = atorvastatin, AT 10 = atorvastatin 10 mg, AT 80 = atorvastatin 80 mg, P = placebo, PR = pravastatin, S = statin. Adapted from: J Am Coll Cardiol 2004;43:2142-6.

26.3%, $p = 0.005$). Patients with intensive lowering of LDL-C plus a reduction in C-reactive protein (decreased vascular inflamation) had the best prognosis (N Engl J Med 2004;350:1495).

b. **TNT.** In this trial, 10,001 men and women with clinically evident CHD and LDL-C < 130 mg/dL were randomized to atorvastatin 10 mg vs. 80 mg. The primary endpoint was death from CHD, nonfatal MI, resuscitation after cardiac arrest, or fatal/nonfatal stroke. At a median follow-up of 4.9 years, atorvastatin 80 mg reduced the primary endpoint by 22% (8.7% vs 10.9%, $p < 0.001$) (N Engl J Med 2005;352:1425-35). Atorvastatin 80 mg also reduced the risk of a major coronary event by 20% ($p = 0.002$), stroke by 23% ($p = 0.007$), hospitalization for heart failure by 26% ($p = 0.01$), and any cardiovascular event by 19% ($p < 0.001$). Mean LDL-C levels were 77 mg/dL with atorvastatin 80 mg vs. 101 mg/dL with atorvastatin 10 mg. Persistently elevated LFTs were more common with atorvastatin 80 mg (1.2% vs. 0.2%, $p < 0.001$), and rhabdomyolysis was rare in both groups (2 and 3 cases in the 80-mg and 10-mg groups, respectively).

c. **IDEAL.** In this trial, 8888 men and women with a history of MI and who qualified for statin therapy by national guidelines at time of recruitment were randomized to atorvastatin 80 mg/d or simvastatin 20 mg/d. Mean baseline LDL-C was 121 mg/dL, and mean on-treatment LDL-C levels were 81 mg/dL (atorvastatin group) and 104 mg/dL (simvastatin group). At a median follow-up of 4.8 years, atorvastatin reduced the primary endpoint of a major coronary event (coronary death, nonfatal MI, resuscitated cardiac arrest) by 11% ($p = 0.07$). Atorvastatin also reduced nonfatal MI by 17% ($p = 0.02$) and major cardiovascular events by 13% ($p = 0.02$). All-cause mortality was not different between treatment groups. Atorvastatin patients had higher rates of drug discontinuation for adverse events and more liver transaminase elevations (1% vs. 0.1% with simvastatin for ALT; 0.4% vs. 0.04% with simvastatin for AST).

d. **Other Trials.** The ongoing Study of the Effectiveness of Additional Reduction of Cholesterol and Homocysteine (SEARCH), which compares simvastatin 80 mg/d vs. 20 mg/d, will further define the role for intensive LDL-C lowering.

3. **Atherosclerosis Imaging Trials.** In the Reversal of Atherosclerosis with Aggressive Lipid Lowering (REVERSAL) trial, pravastatin 40 mg/d (on-treatment LDL-C 110 mg/dL) led to progression of atherosclerosis, whereas atorvastatin 80 mg/d (on-treatment LDL-C 79 mg/dL) did not. Similar results using carotid intima-media thickness as an endpoint were obtained in the Atorvastatin vs. Simvastatin Atherosclerosis Progression (ASAP) and Arterial Biology for the Investigation of the Treatment Effects of Reducing Cholesterol (ARBITER) trials. Most recently, in A Study to Evaluate the Effect of Rosuvastatin on Intravascular Ultrasound-Derived Coronary Atheroma Burden (ASTEROID), rosuvastatin 40 mg led to significant regression of atherosclerosis (Figure 1.5). In ASTEROID, average on-treatment LDL-C was 61 mg/dL (53% reduction in LDL-C), well below the optional goal of < 70 mg/dL suggested by ATP III, and HDL-C was increased by 15%, with a final LDL-C/HDL-C ratio of 1.3. (Neither atorvastatin 80 mg nor rosuvastatin 40 mg are indicated as starting doses for these therapies, and neither agent has an indication in the package insert for stabilization or reversal of atherosclerosis.)

C. Dyslipidemia Trials in Type 2 Diabetes

1. **Statin Trials in Type 2 Diabetes.** Four recent statin trials provide strong support for intensive LDL-C lowering in patients with type 2 diabetes. In CARDS, 2838 patients with type 2 diabetes, no clinical cardiovascular disease (absence of coronary, cerebrovascular, or severe peripheral vascular disease), LDL-C ≤ 160 mg/dL, and at least 1 other risk factor (hypertension, retinopathy, microalbuminuria, macroalbuminuria, current smoking) were randomized to atorvastatin 10 mg/d or placebo. (LDL-C was 119 mg/dL at baseline and 73 mg/dL on atorvastatin treatment.) At 4 years, atorvastatin reduced the first occurrence of any major vascular event by 37% (5.8% vs. 9.0%, $p = 0.001$) (Table 7.1). There was also a 27% reduction in all-cause mortality (borderline statistical significance). The absolute reduction in vascular events was 3.7%, and the number needed to treat x 4 years to prevent one major vascular event was only 27. It was estimated that 4 years of atorvastatin therapy in 1000 CARDS patients would prevent 37 first major cardiovascular events and 50 first or

subsequent events. Benefits were consistent regardless of baseline lipid levels, gender, or age. Atorvastatin was also very well tolerated: there were no cases of rhabdomyolysis and no differences in muscle or liver adverse effects compared to placebo (Lancet 2004;364:685-96). In the diabetes substudy of ASCOT, 2553 type 2 diabetic patients (of 10,305 total patients) with well-controlled hypertension, no CHD, and average cholesterol levels were randomized to atorvastatin 10 mg/d or placebo. At 3.3 years, atorvastatin reduced major cardiovascular events or procedures by 23% (9.2% vs. 11.9%, $p = 0.036$) (Diabetes Care 2005;28:1151-7). Further positive results were demonstrated in the diabetes substudy of HPS, in which 5963 type 2 diabetic subjects (of 20,536 total patients in HPS) were randomized to simvastatin 40 mg/d or placebo. At 5 years, simvastatin reduced the first occurrence of any major vascular event (MI, coronary death, stroke, revascularization) by 22% (20.2% vs. 25.1% for placebo, $p < 0.0001$). There were also highly significant reductions among the 2912 diabetic subjects without occlusive arterial disease at entry (risk reduction 33%, $p = 0.0003$) and among the 2426 subjects with pretreatment LDL-C < 116 mg/dL (risk reduction 27%, $p = 0.0007$) (Lancet 2003;361:2005-16) (Table 7.2). It was estimated that 5 years of simvastatin would prevent 80 major vascular events per 1000 diabetic patients. In a post hoc analysis of 1501 diabetic patients with stable coronary heart disease in the TNT study (p. 87), high-dose (80 mg/d) atorvastatin reduced major cardiovascular events by 25% at 4.9 years compared to atorvastatin 10 mg/d (Table 7.3).

2. **Fibrate Trials in Type 2 Diabetes.** In the Fenofibrate Intervention and Event Lowering in Diabetes (FIELD) study, 9795 patients with type 2 diabetes (including 2131 with previous cardiovascular disease), total cholesterol of 115-250 mg/dL, total cholesterol/HDL-C ratio ≥ 4, and triglycerides of 90-445 mg/dL who were not on statin therapy at baseline were randomized to receive micronized fenofibrate 200 mg/d or placebo. At 1 year, LDL-C was reduced by 12%, HDL-C was increased by 4.5%, and triglycerides were reduced by 30% with fenofibrate compared with placebo. At 5 years, the primary endpoint of coronary events (CHD death or nonfatal MI) was not significantly different between treatment groups (hazard ratio

0.89, 95% CI 0.75-1.05; p = 0.16), but nonfatal MI was reduced by 24% (p = 0.01), coronary revascularization was reduced by 21% (p = 0.003), and total cardiovascular events were reduced by 11% (p = 0.035); microvascular disease, in particular retinopathy, was also reduced (Lancet 2005;366:1849-61). There were no significant reductions in CHD mortality (1.19 [95% CI 0.90–1.57]) or total mortality (1.11 [0.95–1.29]). These results are difficult to apply to clinical practice, however, because FIELD patients were not on statin therapy, as would be expected in clinical practice, and during the trial 17% of placebo patients and 8% of fenofibrate patients began other lipid-lowering therapy, predominantly statins. Additional information is expected from the Action to Control Cardiovascular Risk in Diabetes (ACCORD) trial, in which ~10,000 patients with type 2 diabetes will receive both a fibrate and a statin to examine the effects of combined lowering of LDL-C and triglyceride and raising HDL-C on MI, stroke, and CHD death.

D. Therapeutic Implications. All patients with type 2 diabetes at increased risk for cardiovascular disease should receive statin therapy to reduce LDL-C by a *minimum of 30-40%*, regardless of baseline LDL-C levels. For diabetic patients *without* atherosclerotic vascular disease, NCEP ATP III guidelines recommend a minimum LDL-C target < 100 mg/dL (Circulation 2004;110:227-239). For diabetic patients *with* CHD or other clinical forms of atherosclerosis, the AHA/ACC secondary prevention guidelines state that it is reasonable to treat such patients to an LDL-C < 70 mg/dL (Circulation 2006;113:2363-2372). Use of minimal drug therapy to produce small changes in LDL-C to barely attain LDL-C goal is not recommended. Adjunctive pharmacotherapy is recommended for patients who remain above target LDL-C despite statins. Although studies generally did not include people < 40 years of age, it may be prudent to consider statin therapy in patients with diabetes under the age of 40 if they would have otherwise met criteria for these studies.

Table 7.1. 4-Year Results of the Collaborative Atorvastatin Diabetes Study (CARDS)

	Atorvastatin 10 mg/d (n = 1428)	Placebo (n = 1410)	Relative Risk Reduction
Major vascular events* (%)	5.8	9.0	37%†
Acute coronary events (%)	3.6	5.5	36%
Coronary revascularization (%)	1.7	2.4	31%
Stroke (%)	1.5	2.8	48%

* Acute coronary heart disease death, nonfatal MI, hospitalized unstable angina, resuscitated cardiac arrest, coronary revascularization, stroke

† $p = 0.001$

From: Lancet 2004;364:685-96

Table 7.2. 5-Year Results of the Diabetes Substudy of the Heart Protection Study (HPS)

	Simvastatin 40 mg/d (n = 2978)	Placebo (n = 2985)	p-Value
Major coronary events (%)	9.4	12.6	< 0.0001
Nonfatal MI (%)	3.5	5.5	0.0002
Coronary death (%)	6.5	8.0	0.02
Stroke (%)	5.0	6.5	0.01
Revascularization (%)	8.7	10.4	0.02
Major vascular events* (%)	20.2	25.1	< 0.0001

* Nonfatal MI, coronary death, stroke, or revascularization procedure

From: Lancet 2003;361:2005-16

Table 7.3. 5-Year Results of the Treat to New Targets (TNT) Study in Diabetics: Post-hoc Analysis

	Atorvastatin 80 mg/d (n = 748)	Atorvastatin 10 mg/d (n = 753)	p-Value
Major cardiovascular events* (%)	13.8	17.9	0.026
Major cerebrovascular events (%)	7.0	10.0	0.037

* Death from CHD, nonfatal MI, resuscitated cardiac arrest, or fatal/nonfatal stroke.
From: N Engl J Med 2005;352:1425-35; American Diabetes Association Meeting, June, 2005, San Diego, CA

Goals of Therapy

LDL-C lowering is the primary goal of therapy for patients with type 2 diabetes. Non-HDL-C (LDL-C + VLDL-C), calculated by subtracting HDL-C from total cholesterol, is a secondary goal of therapy after LDL-C lowering in persons with triglycerides ≥ 200 mg/dL. LDL-C and non-HDL-C goals in type 2 diabetic patients are < 100 mg/dL and < 130 mg/dL, respectively; targets < 70 mg/dL and < 100 mg/dL are reasonable for diabetic patients with CHD or other clinical forms of atherosclerosis.

Treatment of Elevated LDL-C

The risk of cardiovascular events in diabetic subjects without CHD is the same as the risk in nondiabetic subjects with CHD (Table 6.2, p. 87), and approximately 80% of diabetic individuals eventually die of a cardiovascular cause. Given the heightened risk of cardiovascular disease conferred by diabetes, the National Cholesterol Education Program Adult Treatment Panel (ATP) III elevated diabetes to a "CHD risk equivalent" and recommended the same LDL-C targets and drug initiation levels for diabetic patients as for individuals with CHD. Based on the results of HPS and other trials, an update from ATP III recommended that all patients with type 2 diabetes at increased risk of cardiovascular disease receive statin therapy to reduce LDL-

C by *at least 30-40%* (Table 7.4) (Circulation 2004;110:227-239). More recently, based on two trials published subsequent to the ATP III update that further support the cardiovascular benefit for intensive LDL lowering — TNT and IDEAL (p. 104) — the AHA/ACC issued a 2006 update to their secondary prevention guidelines stating that it is reasonable to treat patients with CHD or other clinical forms of atherosclerotic disease to an LDL cholesterol < 70 mg/dL (Circulation 2006;113:2363-2372). Use of minimal drug therapy to produce small reductions in LDL-C to barely attain LDL-C goal is not recommended. If LDL-C levels at 6 weeks remain above target, intensification of diet and drugs, including add-on drug therapy, is recommended (Figure 7.5). Difficult-to-control patients should be referred to a lipid specialist.

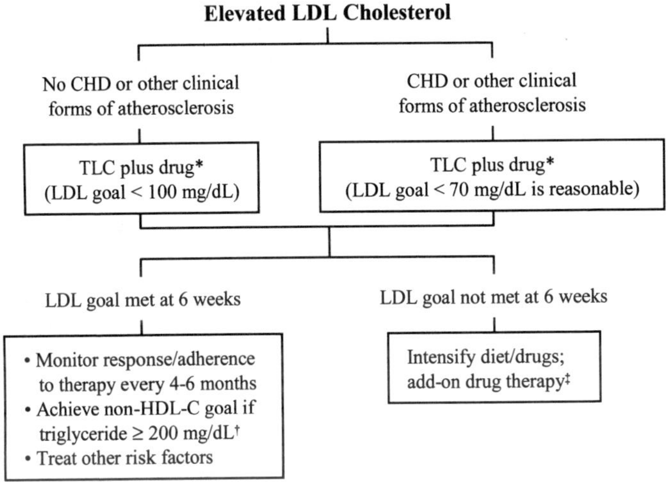

Figure 7.5. Treatment of Elevated LDL-C in Type 2 Diabetes

CHD = coronary heart disease; HDL-C= high-density lipoprotein; LDL-C = low-density lipoprotein; TLC = therapeutic lifestyle changes.

* Initial drug therapy usually consist of standard dose of a statin to reduce LDL-C levels by at least 30-40% (Table 7.4). For patients with CHD or other clinical forms of atherosclerosis, an LDL-C goal < 70 mg/dL is reasonable and frequently requires ≥ 50% reductions in LDL-C levels (Table 7.5). Use of minimal drug therapy to produce small reductions in LDL-C to barely attain LDL-C goal is not recommended.

† For triglyceride levels ≥ 200 mg/dL, non-HDL-C goal is < 130 mg/d. For patients with CHD or other clinical forms of atherosclerosis, a non-HDL-C goal < 100 mg/dL is reasonable. Non-HDL-C = total cholesterol minus HDL-C.

‡ If LDL-C levels at 6 weeks remain above LDL-C target, options include: (1) intensify diet therapy and consider adding plant sterols/stanols 2 gm/day and increasing soluble fiber to 10-25 gm/day; (2) intensify statin therapy; (3) add ezetimibe, a bile acid sequestrant, or niacin; (4) if elevated triglyceride or low HDL-C is present, consider adding niacin, a fibrate, or fish oil to statin therapy. Difficult-to-control patients should be referred to a lipid specialist.

Adapted from: NCEP ATP III update (Circulation 2004;110:227-239), AHA/ACC secondary prevention guideline update (Circulation 2006;113:2363-2372).

Table 7.4. Doses of Statins Required to Attain an Approximate 30-40% Reduction in LDL-C Levels (Standard Doses)*

Drug	Dose (mg/d)	LDL-C Reduction (%)
Rosuvastatin	5-10	39-45
Atorvastatin	10	39
Simvastatin	20-40	35-41
Pravastatin	40	34
Lovastatin	40	31
Fluvastatin	40-80	25-35

Estimated LDL-C reductions were obtained from US Food and Drug Administration package inserts for each drug. For every doubling of the dose above the standard dose, an approximate 6% decrease in LDL-C levels can be obtained. Rosuvastatin is available in doses up to 40 mg; atorvastatin, simvastatin, pravastatin, lovastatin and fluvastatin are available in doses up to 80 mg. From: NCEP ATP III guideline update (Circulation 2004;110:227-239).

* Diabetic patients with established cardiovascular disease are at very high risk of cardiovascular events and frequently require ≥ 50% reductions in LDL-C levels to achieve an LDL-C target < 70 mg/dL (Table 7.5).

Table 7.5. Drug Doses Required to Attain ≥ 50% Reduction in LDL Cholesterol Levels

Drug	Dose (mg/d)	LDL Reduction (%)
Rosuvastatin	20*-40†	52-59
Atorvastatin	80†	51-54
Ezetimibe/simvastatin	10/20‡-10/80†	52-60

Estimated LDL-C reductions obtained from: Am J Cardiol 1998;81:582-7; Am J Cardiol 2003;92:152-60; Mayo Clin Proc 2004;79:620-9; Am Heart J 2004;148:e4.

* Optional starting dose

† Not recommended as starting dose per US Food and Drug Administration package inserts

‡ Recommended usual starting dose

Treatment of Low HDL-C and Elevated Triglyceride

A. **Low HDL-C.** HDL-C is involved in reverse cholesterol transport from the peripheral tissues to the liver. A depressed HDL-C level (< 40 mg/dL) is a powerful predictor of vascular risk. Causes of low HDL-C include elevated triglycerides, obesity, physical inactivity, cigarette smoking, high carbohydrate diets (> 60% of calories), type 2 diabetes, drugs (1st/2nd generation beta-blockers, anabolic steroids, progestational agents), and genetic factors. Nonpharmacologic measures that increase HDL-C include weight loss, exercise, smoking cessation, and low-glycemic diets that are high in monounsaturated fats, omega-3 fats, and lean protein. Alcohol raises HDL-C levels but is not recommended for that purpose. Once LDL-C and non-HDL-C goals are met, drug therapy to raise HDL-C may be considered for higher-risk individuals (Figure 7.6). ATP III does not establish a goal for HDL-C, but the American Heart Association recommends initiation of niacin or fibrate therapy in women with HDL-C < 50 mg/dL (Circulation 2004;109:672-93). The American Diabetes Association recommends an HDL-C level > 40 mg/dL (noting that an HDL-C > 50 mg/dL has been advocated in women), and suggests the use of a fibrate, niacin, or combination therapy with statin plus either fibrate or niacin to raise HDL-C levels (Diabetes Care 2006;29:S4-42). TZD's will also raise HDL-C levels in type 2 diabetes.

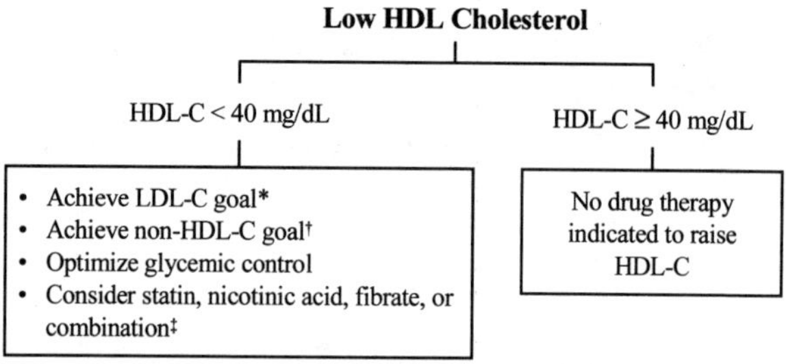

Figure 7.6. Treatment of Low HDL-C in Type 2 Diabetes

* LDL-C goal < 100 mg/dL; for patients with CHD or other clinical forms of atherosclerosis, it is reasonable to treat LDL-C to < 70 mg/dL (Circulation 2006;113:2363-2372). When indicated, drug therapy (statins preferred) should be used to reduce LDL-C by at least 30-40%.

† Non-HDL-C is a secondary goal of therapy after LDL-C lowering for persons with triglycerides ≥ 200 mg/dL. Non-HDL-C goal is < 130 mg/dL; for patients with CHD or other clinical forms of atherosclerosis, it is reasonable to treat non-HDL-C to < 100 mg/dL. Non-HDL-C = total cholesterol minus HDL-C.

‡ Monitor for worsening glycemic control (niacin) and for myopathy/rhabdomyolysis, especially with statin/fibrate or statin/niacin combination therapy. Fenofibrate has less risk of complications in combination therapy and is therefore the preferred fibrate.

B. Elevated Triglyceride. Elevated triglyceride is an independent risk factor for coronary disease and is associated with atherogenic VLDL-C remnants and small dense LDL-C particles, which correlate with the extent and progression of atherosclerosis. ATP III defines normal triglyceride as < 150 mg/dL, borderline-high triglyceride as 150-199 mg/dL, high triglyceride as 200-499 mg/dL, and very high triglyceride as ≥ 500 mg/dL. Since remnant lipoproteins are comprised of partially degraded VLDL-C particles, elevated VLDL-C levels can be used as a marker for the presence of remnant lipoproteins and elevated risk. ATP III recognizes non-HDL-C (LDL-C + VLDL-C) as a secondary target of therapy in patients with high triglyceride (≥ 200 mg/dL) and sets the non-HDL-C goal at 30 mg/dL higher than the LDL-C goal (i.e., < 100 mg/dL in diabetics), based on the assumption that higher VLDL-C levels are associated with remnant lipoproteins and increased vascular risk. Non-HDL-C is determined by subtracting HDL-C from total cholesterol. Causes of elevated triglyceride include lifestyle-related causes (obesity, physical inactivity, cigarette smoking, excess alcohol intake, high carbohydrate diet), other secondary causes (diabetes mellitus, chronic renal failure, nephrotic syndrome, Cushing's disease, lipodystrophy, pregnancy, various drugs), and genetic causes. The potential benefits of lowering triglyceride levels are not as well studied as those of lowering LDL-C. For triglyceride levels of 150-199 mg/dL, emphasis is placed on therapeutic lifestyle changes, glycemic control, omega-3 fats, and LDL-C lowering; drug therapy to reduce triglycerides is not recommended (Figure 7.7). For triglyceride levels of 200-499 mg/dL, primary therapy is directed at LDL-C lowering, and non-HDL-C is a secondary goal of therapy. Drug therapy may be considered in high-risk patients to achieve the non-HDL-C goal. Pharmacologic approaches include intensification of LDL-lowering therapy and/or the addition of omega-3 fats or nicotinic acid or fibrates, when used with appropriate caution. For very high triglyceride levels (≥ 500 mg/dL), the primary goal of therapy is to prevent acute pancreatitis by rapidly lowering triglycerides to < 500 mg/dL with marked restriction of processed carbohydrates (i.e., avoidance of processed foods and drinks containing sugars or starches), weight reduction, increased physical activity, and the use of either a fibrate or nicotinic acid along with omega-3 fats. Once triglycerides are < 500 mg/dL, attention is directed toward achieving LDL-C and non-HDL-C targets.

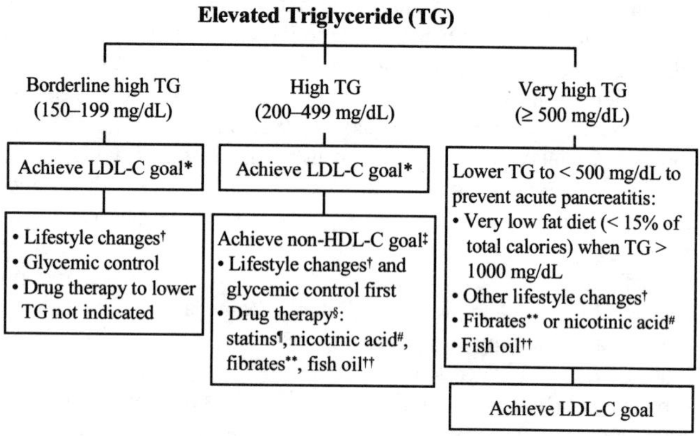

Figure 7.7. Treatment of Elevated Triglyceride in Type 2 Diabetes

* LDL-C goal < 100 mg/dL; for patients with CHD or other clinical forms of atherosclerosis, it is reasonable to treat LDL-C to < 70 mg/dL. When indicated, drug therapy (statins preferred) should be used to lower LDL-C by at least 30-40%.

† Weight control, increased physical activity, smoking cessation, restriction of alcohol in some, avoidance of high-carbohydrate diets (> 60% of total calories), discontinuation of nonessential drugs that raise cholesterol.

‡ Non-HDL-C goal < 130 mg/dL; for patients with CHD or other clinical forms of atherosclerosis, it is reasonable to treat non-HDL-C to < 100 mg/dL.

§ May need high-dose statin or moderate-dose statin plus either nicotinic acid or fibrate

¶ Statins lower triglycerides by 7-30% (20-50% or higher in patients with severely elevated triglyceride).

Nicotinic acid lowers triglycerides by 20-50%, but doses ≥ 2 gm/d can worsen hyperglycemia in persons with diabetes or insulin resistance.

** Fibrates lower triglycerides by 20-50% but can raise LDL-C in patients with hypertriglyceridemia. Fibrates are the best choice for acute reductions in triglycerides when used with appropriate caution.

†† Omega-3 fats (EPA + DHA) (3-4 gm/d) reduce triglycerides by 20-45% and are useful adjuncts to statin therapy. Omacor, which contains highly purified omega-3 ethyl esters (EPA, DHA), has been approved by the FDA for the treatment of triglycerides ≥ 500 mg/dL; the dose in clinical studies was 4 gm/day.

Drug Therapy for Dyslipidemia

Drug therapy plays a central role in the management of dyslipidemia, improving lipid profile, slowing the progression of atherosclerosis, stabilizing rupture-prone plaques, reducing the risk of arterial thrombosis, and improving prognosis. For patients who require drug therapy, the drug should be added to, not substituted for, diet therapy and lifestyle modification. Table 7.6 lists effective cholesterol-lowering drugs.

A. **Statin Therapy.** Statins are overwhelmingly the drug class of choice for improving dyslipidemia and cardiovascular prognosis in type 2 diabetes. In addition to lowering LDL-C levels by 18-55%, statins lower the number of small, dense LDL-C particles, raise HDL-C levels by 5-15%, and lower triglycerides by 7-30%. The recent update to the National Cholesterol Education Program Adult Treatment Panel (ATP) III recommends that all type 2 diabetic patients at increased risk for cardiovascular disease should receive statin therapy to reduce LDL-C by *at least 30-40%*, regardless of baseline LDL-C levels (Table 7.4). A minimum LDL-C target < 100 mg/dL is recommended (Circulation 2004;110:227-239). Similar recommendations were published in guidelines from the American College of Physicians (ACP) (Ann Intern Med 2004;140:644-9). More recently, based on two trials published subsequent to the ATP III update that further support the cardiovascular benefit for intensive LDL lowering — TNT and IDEAL (p. 104) — the AHA/ACC issued a 2006 update to their secondary prevention guidelines stating that it is reasonable to treat diabetic patients with CHD or other clinical forms of atherosclerotic disease to an LDL-C < 70 mg/dL (Circulation 2006;113:2363-2372). The role of statin therapy in lower-risk patients with type 2 diabetes (e.g., younger patients with LDL-C < 130 mg/dL and no other cardiovascular risk factors) awaits definition. (See Table 7.6 for contraindications and adverse effects.)

B. **Adjuncts to Statin Therapy.** Statin monotherapy may not achieve LDL-C goal or completely normalize the lipid profile in type 2 diabetes, and adjunctive pharmacotherapy may be required.

   1. **Ezetimibe.** Ezetimibe is a newer agent that inhibits the absorption of cholesterol and phytosterols from the small intestine. When used as monotherapy, ezetimibe lowers LDL-C by 18%. When added to

statin therapy, ezetimibe 10 mg/d further reduces LDL-C by 25%, triglycerides by 10-15% and C-reactive protein by 10%, and raises HDL-C levels (Circulation 2003;107:2409-15, J Am Coll Cardiol 2002;40:2125-34, Am J Cardiol 2002;90:1084-91). (By comparison, each doubling of statin dose provides about 6% additional LDL-C reduction.) The combination of ezetimibe and statin is safe, effective and well tolerated, and is particularly helpful in the many diabetic patients who require ≥ 50% reductions in LDL-C levels. Ezetimibe in combination with simvastatin is available as a single tablet (Vytorin) is doses of 10/10 mg, 10/20 mg, 10/40 mg, and 10/80 mg.

2. **Niacin.** Niacin will raise HDL-C by 15-35% and lower LDL-C by 10-25%, triglycerides by 20-50%, and lipoprotein(a) by 20-30%. Niacin also improves prothrombotic tendencies by reducing plasminogen activator inhibitor-1 (PAI-1), fibrinogen, and alpha-2 antiplasmin levels. Niacin (and fibrates) can shift small, dense LDL-C particles toward larger, more buoyant particles, which may be less atherogenic. However, niacin can worsen insulin resistance, impair glucose tolerance, and raise HbA_{1c} levels in some diabetics, and there is an increased risk of myopathy/rhabdomyolysis when niacin is used, particularly at higher doses, in conjunction with a statin. When niacin is administered, lower doses (e.g., Niaspan < 1.5 gm/d) and glucose monitoring are recommended . Flushing can be decreased/prevented by taking aspirin 30-60 minutes prior to the dose.
3. **Omega-3 fatty acids.** Omega-3 fats, usually in the form of concentrated fish oil, are useful for diabetic dyslipidemia. Low doses (1-1.5 gm/d) have been shown to reduce cardiovascular mortality, primarily by reducing sudden death; higher doses (3-4 gm/d) can lower triglycerides by 20-50% and are well-tolerated adjuncts to statins. Omacor, which contains highly purified omega-3 ethyl esters (85% EPA + DHA), is approved for the treatment of triglycerides ≥ 500 mg/dL; the dose in clinical studies was 4 gm/day.
4. **Fibrates.** Fibrates improve the lipid profile in diabetic dyslipidemia by lowering triglycerides by 20-50%, raising HDL-C by 16-35%, and shifting small, dense LDL-C particles to larger, less atherogenic particles. However, the risk for myopathy and rhabdomyolysis is increased when fibrates are used with statins, with the possible exception of fenofibrate (Drug Metab Dispos 2002;30:1280-7).

Table 7.6. Effective Lipid-Modifying Drug Therapy

Drug (usual starting/max dose)	Lipid Effects	Comments
HMG-CoA Reductase Inhibitors (Statins)		
Atorvastatin (10/80 mg/d) Fluvastatin (40/80 mg/d) Lovastatin (20/80 mg/d) Pravastatin (20/80 mg/d) Rosuvastatin (5/40 mg/d) Simvastatin (20/80 mg/d)	LDL-C: ↓ 18-55% HDL-C: ↑ 5-15% TG: ↓ 7-30%	*Major use:* Overwhelmingly the drug class of choice for elevated LDL-C levels. Highly effective for lowering LDL-C and preventing cardiovascular and cerebrovascular events. *Absolute CI:* active or chronic liver disease, pregnancy, lactation. *Relative CI:* concomitant use of cyclosporine, macrolide antibiotics, various antifungal drugs, cytochrome P-450 inhibitors; previous intolerance to statins due to myalgias, elevated liver transaminases, other side effects. *Adverse effects:* myopathy, ↑ liver transaminases. Fibrates and nicotinic acid should be used with caution in combination with statins.
Cholesterol Absorption Inhibitor		
Ezetimibe (10 mg/d)	LDL-C: ↓ 18 (as monotherapy); further ↓ by 25% when added to statins HDL-C: ↑ 1% TG: ↓ 8%	*Major use:* Safe, effective, and well-tolerated adjunct to statins when further LDL-C lowering is required. Not recommended in moderate or severe hepatic insufficiency. Effectiveness reduced when given within 2-4 hours of bile acid sequestrant. *CI:* combination with statin in patients with active liver disease or unexplained persistent transaminase elevations. *Adverse effects:* GI complaints.

↑ = increases, ↓ = decreases, CI = contraindication, HDL-C= HDL cholesterol, LDL = LDL cholesterol, Lp(a) = lipoprotein(a), TG = triglyceride

Table 7.6. Effective Lipid-Modifying Drug Therapy

Drug (usual starting/max dose)	Lipid Effects	Comments
Nicotinic Acid (Niacin)		
Immediate-release form (50 mg/4.5 gm/d) Sustained-release form (500 mg/2 gm/d) Extended-release form (500 mg/2 gm/d)	LDL-C: ↓ 5-25% HDL-C: ↑ 15-35% TG: ↓ 20-50%	*Major use:* Useful in nearly all dyslipidemias. Uniquely effective in atherogenic dyslipidemia. Also useful for elevated Lp(a) levels and as adjunctive therapy for mixed dyslipidemia. *Absolute CI:* chronic liver disease, severe gout. *Relative CI:* hyperuricemia, high doses (> 3 gm/d) in type 2 diabetes. Caution in active liver or peptic ulcer disease, hyperuricemia, gout. *Adverse effects:* flushing, hyperglycemia, hyperuricemia/gout, upper GI distress, hepatotoxicity (esp. sustained-release).
Bile Acid Sequestrants		
Colesevelam (3.8/4.4 gm/d) Cholestyramine ([4-16]/24 gm/d) Colestipol ([5-20]/30 gm/d)	LDL-C: ↓ 15-30% HDL-C: ↑ 3-5% TG: usually not affected; may ↑	*Major use:* Moderate hypercholesterolemia, younger patients with elevated LDL-C, and women with elevated LDL-C who are considering pregnancy (sequestrants are not absorbed out of the GI tract and lack systemic toxicity). Also useful as adjunctive therapy with statins. *Absolute CI:* familial dysbetalipoproteinemia, triglyceride > 400 mg/dL. *Relative CI:* triglyceride > 200 mg/dL. *Adverse effects:* GI complaints common, decreased absorption of several drugs.

↑ = increases, ↓ = decreases, CI = contraindication, HDL-C= HDL cholesterol, LDL-C = LDL cholesterol, Lp(a) = lipoprotein(a), TG = triglyceride

Table 7.6. Effective Lipid-Modifying Drug Therapy

Drug (usual starting/max dose)	Lipid Effects	Comments
Fibric Acid Derivatives		
Gemfibrozil (600 mg bid) Fenofibrate (130-200 mg/d) Clofibrate (1000 mg bid)	LDL-C: ↓ 5-20% (may ↑ LDL-C if ↑ TG at baseline) HDL-C: ↑ 10-35% TG: ↓ 20-50%	*Major uses:* Hypertriglyceridemia, atherogenic dyslipidemia (especially in type 2 diabetes). *Absolute CI:* severe hepatic or renal dysfunction, primary biliary cirrhosis, gallbladder disease. *Relative CI:* combined therapy with statins (occasional occurrence of severe myopathy or rhabdomyolysis). Use with caution when combining with coumarin anticoagulants or cyclosporine. *Adverse effects:* dyspepsia, upper GI complaints, cholesterol gallstones, myopathy.
Omega-3 Fatty Acids (Fish Oil)		
Omega-3 acid ethyl esters (4 gm/d)	TG: ↓ 45% non-HDL-C: ↓ 14% LDL-C: ↑ 44% HDL-C: ↑ 9%	*Major use:* Hypertriglyceridemia (TG ≥500 mg/dL). *CI:* Use with caution in patients with known hypersensitivity or allergy to fish, and in women who are pregnant or breastfeeding. *Adverse effects:* eructation, dyspepsia, taste perversion.

↑ = increases, ↓ = decreases, CI = contraindication, HDL-C= HDL cholesterol, LDL-C = LDL cholesterol, Lp(a) = lipoprotein(a), TG = triglyceride

Chapter 8

Control of Hypertension in Type 2 Diabetes

Hypertension affects 50 million Americans and 1 billion individuals worldwide, including approximately 2 out of 3 persons with type 2 diabetes. Twelve percent of Americans have both diabetes and hypertension, and approximately 75% of persons with type 2 diabetes have hypertension (Am J Prev Med 2002;22:42-48, J Am Geriatr Soc 2001;49:109–16, Diabetes Care 1998;21:1414–31). The prevalence of hypertension is 2-fold higher and the incidence of cardiovascular events is 6-fold higher in diabetic patients compared to nondiabetic age-matched subjects (Diabetes Care 2005;28:Suppl 1, Arch Intern Med 1989;149:1942–5, JAMA 1967;202:104–10). Numerous epidemiological and observational studies demonstrate a direct, continuous relationship between increasing blood pressure and vascular risk, with no apparent lower threshold (although data are lacking below a blood pressure of 115/75 mmHg) (Lancet 2002;360:1903-1913, J Hypertens 2000;18:1193-1196). Systolic, diastolic, mean arterial, and pulse pressures all predict vascular risk, although systolic and diastolic blood pressures are recommended as the best means of classifying blood pressure (Circulation 2005;111:697-716). Among individuals aged 55-65 years without hypertension at baseline, the residual lifetime risk of developing hypertension is 90% (JAMA 2002;287:1003-10).

More than 90% of hypertension is idiopathic (essential), while 5-10% can be ascribed to an identifiable cause (secondary hypertension). Essential hypertension is caused by increased vascular reactivity and/or inappropriate renal retention of salt and water. Diabetic subjects are especially prone to these problems due to a hyperactive renin-angiotensin-aldosterone system and increased sympathetic tone. In addition, hyperglycemia increases salt and water retention since, for every molecule of glucose filtered and reabsorbed in the kidney, one molecule of sodium is also absorbed. Over many years, this leads to accelerated atherosclerosis in large vessels, obliterative changes and/or thinning and rupture of small vessels, and increased workload on the heart. Intensive treatment of hypertension in diabetic patients reduces by 30% the incidence of and fatality from coronary heart disease, stroke, heart failure, and kidney disease. Blood pressure control also reduces the progression of diabetic retinopathy and deterioration in visual acuity (BMJ 1998;317:703-13).

Hypertension is grossly underdiagnosed and undertreated. Results from the Third National Health and Nutrition Evaluation Survey (NHANES III) indicated that 29% of diabetic individuals with hypertension were unaware of the diagnosis; 43% of diabetic individuals with hypertension were untreated; 55% of treated diabetic individuals had a blood pressure ≥ 140/90 mmHg; and only 12% of treated diabetic individuals had a blood pressure < 130/85 mmHg (Am J Rev Med 2002;22:42-48). Using NHANES III data, it was estimated that proper control of hypertension could prevent 19-56% and 31-57% of coronary events in men and women, respectively (Am Heart 2003;145:888-895).

Diagnosis of Hypertension

Blood pressure targets for diabetic patients are lower than for the general population. Hypertension in a diabetic patient is defined by a systolic BP ≥ 130 mmHg or a diastolic BP ≥ 80 mmHg, based on the average of two or more readings at two or more visits after the initial screen. (In JNC 7, for the general population, hypertension is defined by a BP ≥ 140/90 mmHg.) A single recording may be sufficient if systolic blood pressure is ≥ 210 mmHg or diastolic blood pressure is ≥ 120 mmHg, especially if symptoms are present, but even very high elevations in blood pressure may occur transiently during extreme stress or acute illness.

Treatment of Diabetic Hypertension

A. **Overview.** Cardiovascular events are 2-4–fold higher in diabetic hypertensives compared to nondiabetic hypertensives, and aggressive blood pressure lowering is recommended in all diabetic subjects to reduce the risk of cardiovascular events, retinopathy, and nephropathy. In the United Kingdom Diabetes Prevention Study (UKPDS) epidemiological study, each 10-mmHg reduction in mean systolic BP decreased the risk of diabetes-related death by 15%, MI by 11%, and microvascular complications by 13% (BMJ 1998;317:703-13). In the Hypertension Optimum Treatment (HOT) study, there was a 51% reduction in cardiovascular events for diabetic patients assigned to a diastolic BP target of 80 mmHg versus a target of 90 mmHg (Lancet 1998;351: 1755-62). Based on these and other data, the Seventh Report of the Joint National Committee on Prevention, Detection, Evaluation, and Treatment of High Blood Pressure (JNC 7) recommends a target BP level of < 130/80 mmHg in patients with type 2 diabetes (JAMA 2003;289:2560-72). This goal has been endorsed by the ADA and the AACE/ACE. The National Kidney Foundation has set a BP goal ≤ 125/75 mmHg for individuals with diabetic nephropathy. Treating to BP ≤ 120/75 mmHg may be even more effective at halting the progression of renal disease and vascular complications, especially for persons with proteinuria > 1 gm/d (Endocr Pract 2006;12:193-222).

B. **Blood Pressure Goals.** In the setting of type 2 diabetes, the goal of therapy is to reduce BP to < 130/80 mmHg. Optimal BP is ≤ 120/75 mmHg. To achieve maximum benefit, systolic and diastolic BP should be reduced to established targets and, based on recent data, rapid lowering of BP is important to reduce MI and stroke (see next page). Despite marked benefits of antihypertensive therapy, only 12% of diabetic patients in the U.S. are well controlled (BP < 130/80 mmHg) (Am J Rev Med 2002;22:42-8).

C. **Therapeutic Lifestyle Changes (Chapter 4).** Therapeutic lifestyle changes should be initiated simultaneously with drug therapy for diabetic patients with systolic BP ≥ 130 mmHg. Measures advocated by JNC 7 include: weight control; limit alcohol to no more than 2 drinks/day (1 oz or 30 mL of ethanol [24 oz beer, 10 oz wine, or 3 oz 80-proof whiskey]) in most men and no more than 1 drink/day in women and lighter-weight persons; increase aerobic physical activity to 30-45 minutes most days of the week; reduce sodium intake to ≤ 100 mmol/d (2.4 gm/d sodium or 6 gm/d sodium chloride); maintain adequate intake of dietary potassium (approximately 90 mmol/d), calcium, magnesium; smoking cessation for overall cardiovascular health; and increase dietary intake of fruits, vegetables, and low-fat dairy and reduce intake of saturated fat and total fat.

D. Initial Drug Therapy. The average diabetic patient with hypertension requires 3.2 drugs to achieve/maintain target BP, with each antihypertensive agent lowering the systolic BP by approximately 10-15 mmHg. In the absence of contraindications, and based on the proven cardioprotective/renoprotective properties of ARB's and ACE inhibitors in diabetic patients, initial therapy with an ARB or ACE inhibitor in combination with a low-dose thiazide diuretic (e.g., hydrochlorothiazide 12.5 mg/d) is a reasonable approach (Figure 8.1). For individuals with chronic renal insufficiency (GFR < 50 mL/min), a loop diuretic should be used instead of a thiazide diuretic. Addition of a diuretic will potentiate the antihypertensive effects of ARB's and ACE inhibitors and offset their tendency to induce hyperkalemia. If monotherapy is employed, an ARB or ACE inhibitor is recommended, followed, if necessary, by a thiazide diuretic. (Consider doubling the usual starting dose of an ACE inhibitor or ARB if the patient is African American.) A beta-blocker or a calcium antagonist may also be considered for second-line therapy, but these agents are commonly reserved for the more than 50% of diabetic patients who require additional drug therapy after an ARB (or ACE inhibitor) and diuretic. Recent hypertension guidelines from AACE identify a BP goal ≤ 130/80 for individuals with diabetes (≤ 120/75 mmHg for proteinuria ≥ 1 gm/d) and recommend an ARB or ACE inhibitor as a first- or second-line agent, a thiazide diuretic (at low-dose with potassium replacement or a potassium-sparing diuretic) as a first- or second-line agent, a beta blocker (preferably one with alpha-blockade, e.g., carvedilol) as a second- or third-line agent, and a calcium antagonist (preferably a nondihydropyridine) as a second-, third-, or fourth-line agent (Endocr Pract 2006;12:193-222). Once-daily, fixed-dose combination drug therapy (e.g., ARB or ACE in combination with a diuretic) may improve patient compliance by minimizing pill burden. Low-dose aspirin, recommended for most type 2 diabetic patients, may further reduce blood pressure when administered before bedtime (J Am Coll Cardiol 2005;46:975-83). Each antihypertensive agent can be expected to lower the systolic blood pressure by about 10-15 mmHg. Patients should be encouraged to record and report home blood pressure measurements to assess the effectiveness of antihypertensive drug therapy and to detect white-coat and reverse white-coat hypertension.

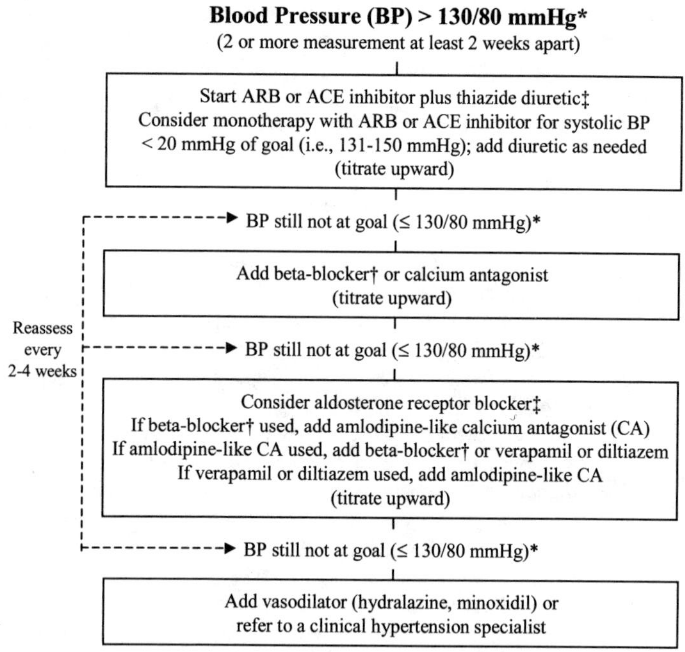

Figure 8.1. Treatment of Diabetic Hypertension

ACE = angiotensin converting enzyme, ARB = angiotensin II receptor blocker.

* BP goal is ≤ 125/75 mmHg for nephropathy plus proteinuria > 1 gm/day. Treat systolic and diastolic BP to goal. Drug therapy should be initiated concurrently with smoking cessation, weight control, physical activity. Most diabetic patients require at least 2 drugs to control BP and many require 3 or more. Check for postural hypotension prior to adjustments in drug therapy. Home BP recordings are recommended to optimize therapy

† Based on GEMINI (p. 131), carvedilol substantially lowers BP when used with an ACE inhibitor and does not worsen insulin resistance or glycemic control

‡ For chronic renal insufficiency (GFR < 50 mL/min), substitute a loop diuretic (e.g., furosemide BID or torsemide QD) for a thiazide diuretic; only use aldosterone receptor blocker if K^+ < 4.8 mEq/L on ARB or ACE inhibitor

E. **Rapidity of Blood Pressure Lowering and Intensification of Drug Therapy.** Recent data indicate important cardiovascular benefits for rapid control of blood pressure. In VALUE, 15,245 high-risk hypertensive patients (32% with type 2 diabetes) were randomized to valsartan or amlodipine. Controlled BP at 6 months was associated with a 25% reduction in fatal and nonfatal cardiac events ($p < 0.05$), with benefits as early as 1 month for immediate responders (Lancet 2004;363:2049-51, Lancet 2004;363:2022-31). Therefore, if BP remains ≥ 130 mmHg at 2 weeks after initial therapy, drug dosages should be optimized or drugs from different drug classes should be added at 3-4–week intervals. A beta-blocker, preferably one with alpha-1 blockade (e.g., carvedilol), which does not increase insulin resistance or worsen hyperglycemia, or a calcium antagonist (e.g., amlodipine, verapamil, diltiazem) is an excellent option for diabetic patients who require additional drug therapy to lower blood pressure after an ARB (or ACE inhibitor) and diuretic. An aldosterone receptor blocker (spironolactone, eplerenone) and/or a centrally-acting vasodilator (hydralazine, minoxidil) may be useful if further drug therapy is required; with an aldosterone receptor blocker, monitoring for hyperkalemia should be performed on days 3, 10, and 21 of therapy. Before proceeding to each successive treatment step, potential reasons for lack of responsiveness should be identified, including pseudohypertension, nonadherence to therapy, volume overload, drug-related causes, and secondary causes of hypertension such as hyperaldosteronism, which can be diagnosed with an elevated aldosterone-to-renin ratio and responds well to anti-aldosterone drugs such as spironolactone and eplerenone. Hospitalization should be considered for patients with BP ≥ 200/120 mmHg and symptomatic target organ damage.

Use of Specific Drug Therapy

A. **ACE Inhibitors.** ACE inhibitors improve event-free survival in patients with atherosclerotic vascular disease, systolic heart failure, asymptomatic left ventricular (LV) dysfunction, or acute myocardial infarction (Circulation 2005;112:1339-1346, Lancet 2003;362:782–8, N Engl J

Med 2000;342:145–53, Lancet 2000;355:1575–81, Circulation 1995;92:3132–7). They also exert renoprotective effects in type 1 diabetes and have been shown to reduce proteinuria and progression to overt nephropathy in type 2 diabetes (Lancet 2000;35:253–9), although a specific renoprotective effect beyond blood pressure lowering in pre-existing diabetic nephropathy has been questioned (Lancet 2005;366:2026-2033). A recent meta-analysis found that ACE inhibitors reduced the incidence of newly diagnosed type 2 diabetes by 27% (J Am Coll Cardiol 2005;46:821-6), although no drug has yet been approved for the prevention of diabetes. Antihypertensive effects usually become apparent within one week and are augmented by the addition of a low-dose thiazide diuretic (e.g., hydrochlorothiazide 12.5 mg). Cough develops in 10%-20% of patients receiving ACE inhibitors and may require discontinuation of therapy. These patients can usually be switched to an ARB without recurrence of cough. Approximately 0.5% of patients (the percentage is higher in African Americans) receiving ACE inhibitors develop angioneurotic edema. ACE inhibitors should be immediately discontinued if symptoms develop, and switching to an ARB does not decrease the risk of this potentially life-threatening complication. Diabetic patients receiving ACE inhibitors should not be treated routinely with potassium supplement or potassium-sparing diuretics, especially if renal insufficiency is present, due to the increased risk of hyperkalemia. Intravascular volume depletion should be corrected (e.g., withholding diuretics or increasing salt intake for several days) before initiating therapy to reduce the risk of symptomatic hypotension. ACE inhibitors should not be used during pregnancy (category D for second and third trimesters; category C for first trimester), and when pregnancy is detected, ACE inhibitors should be discontinued as soon as possible.

B. **Angiotensin Receptor Blockers (ARB's).** ARB's are effective antihypertensive agents with proven cardioprotective properties in patients with hypertensive LVH, heart failure, and acute MI (Lancet 2002;359;995-1003, Lancet 2003;362:772-6, N Engl J Med 2003;349:1893-906). They also exert renoprotective effects, reducing proteinuria and slowing the deterioration in renal function in diabetic nephropathy, as measured by occurrence of doubling of serum creatinine or end-stage renal disease (need for dialysis or renal transplantation)(N Engl J Med 2001;345:861-9, N Engl J Med 2001;345:851-60, N Engl J Med 2001;345:870-8), although a specific renoprotective effect beyond blood pressure lowering in patients with pre-existing diabetic nephropathy has been questioned (Lancet 2005;366:2026-2033). In the LIFE trial, losartan reduced the risk of the composite endpoint of death, MI, or stroke to a greater extent than atenolol in hypertensive patients with LVH (Lancet 2002;359;995-1003). A recent meta-analysis found that ARB's reduced the incidence of newly diagnosed type 2 diabetes by 23% (J Am Coll Cardiol 2005;46:821-6), although no drug has yet been approved for the prevention of diabetes. ARB's are very well tolerated, with an overall incidence of adverse effects similar to placebo. Antihypertensive effects usually become apparent within one week and are augmented by the addition of a low-dose thiazide diuretic (e.g., hydrochlorothiazide 12.5 mg). Most patients who experience a persistent dry cough in response to an ACE inhibitor can be switched to an ARB without recurrence of cough. Diabetic patients receiving ARB's should not be treated routinely with potassium supplement or potassium-sparing diuretics, especially if renal insufficiency is present, due to the risk of hyperkalemia. Intravascular volume depletion should be corrected (e.g., withholding diuretics or increasing salt intake for several days) before initiating therapy to reduce the risk of symptomatic hypotension. Patients who experience angioneurotic edema with an ACE inhibitor are at high risk for this potentially life-threatening complication with ARB's. ARB's should not be used during pregnancy (category D for 2nd/3rd trimesters; category C for 1st trimester); when pregnancy is detected, ARB's should be discontinued.

C. **Renin Inhibitors.** Pharmacological inhibition of the renin-angiotensin system (RAS) via ACE inhibitors and ARB's have been proven to reduce morbidity and mortality in diabetic patients with hypertension, atherosclerosis, nephropathy, and heart failure. The direct renin inhibitor aliskiren has been developed as an alternative means of blocking the RAS. Aliskiren has been shown to lower blood pressure and to be equally effective in diabetic and non-diabetic patients (Pharmacokinet 2006;45:1125-34).

D. **Diuretics.** Diuretics are effective first-line agents in general population studies. However, when treating patients with diabetes they should be used as second-line therapy or as part of combination therapy with an ARB or ACE inhibitor to potentiate blood pressure lowering. Low-dose hydrochlorothiazide in fixed-dose combination with an ARB or ACE inhibitor is often used as first-line therapy in diabetic patients. Recommended starting and maximal doses for diuretics are the equivalent of 12.5 mg and 25 mg of hydrochlorothiazide, respectively. Higher doses increase insulin resistance, worsen glycemic control, lower HDL cholesterol, and increase triglyceride and uric acid levels. In ALLHAT, use of chlorthalidone in doses equivalent to 50 mg hydrochlorothiazide resulted in 30% more individuals being diagnosed with diabetes compared to amlodipine or lisinopril (JAMA 2002;288:2981-97, JAMA 2000;283;1967-75). For individuals with chronic renal insufficiency (GFR < 50 mL/min), a loop diuretic should be used instead of a thiazide diuretic. The major antihypertensive response to diuretics is seen within 1-2 weeks of starting therapy or adjusting the dose. Patients with moderate renal insufficiency and volume-dependant hypertension who do not response to thiazides may require a loop diuretic (furosemide, bumetanide), a high-potency diuretic (metolazone, indapamide, or the longer-acting torsemide), or a combination of metolazone plus a loop diuretic. Potassium-sparing diuretics should generally be avoided in diabetic patients with renal insufficiency and in those receiving potassium supplements, ACE inhibitors, or ARB's.

E. **Beta Blockers.** Type 2 diabetes disrupts normal autonomic balance, predisposing to excessive sympathetic tone and increasing the risk of hypertension, coronary disease, and sudden cardiac death. Diabetic patients have a 3-fold increased risk of sudden death compared to nondiabetic patients. First and second generation beta blockers may worsen insulin resistance, mask symptoms of hypoglycemia, and induce peripheral vasoconstriction, which can worsen peripheral arterial disease in the diabetic patient. Nevertheless, they are effective antihypertensive agents with proven benefits on survival following acute MI and in stable systolic heart failure. They also reduce cardiovascular events at least as well (and possibly better) in diabetic patients as they do in nondiabetic patients, including a 50% reduction in sudden death. Beta blockers are recommended for diabetic patients who require additional drug therapy to lower blood pressure after an ARB (or ACE inhibitor) and diuretic. Beta blockers with alpha-1 blockade, such as carvedilol, are particularly useful in diabetic patients: the 7% alpha-1 blockade is enough to lower insulin resistance, and the resulting difference in insulin sensitivity when carvedilol is compared with a 1st or 2nd generation beta blocker is equivalent to that seen with a thiazolidinedione. The improvement in insulin resistance seen with alpha-1 blockade is due to vasodilation of the vascular bed in muscle, which is an advantage to the diabetic patient. Since insulin resistance and hypertensive ventricular remodeling in type 2 diabetes start long before the development of heart failure, early use of beta blockers to reverse remodeling will benefit the diabetic patient. Among 3029 patients with chronic heart failure randomized to carvedilol or metoprolol in the COMET trial, carvedilol reduced all-cause mortality by 15% (34% vs. 40%, $p = 0.0017$) and new diabetes by 22% at 4.8 years (Lancet 2003;362:7-13). In GEMINI, 1235 patients with type 2 diabetes and hypertension receiving a renin-angiotensin-system blocker (ACE inhibitor or ARB) were randomized to carvedilol 6.25-25 mg twice daily or metoprolol 50-200 mg twice daily. At 35 weeks, carvedilol resulted in better glycemic control (HbA_{1c} levels stabilized with carvedilol but increased with metoprolol), improved insulin sensitivity (insulin resistance was reduced by carvedilol but increased with metoprolol), and less progression to microabluminuria (JAMA 2004;292:2227-36) (Table 8.1). Beta blockers with alpha-1 blockade are generally well tolerated; however, due to alpha-1 blockade, the risk of postural hypotension is increased, and concomitant use of phosphodiesterase inhibitors such as sildenafil (Viagra), tadalafil (Cialis), and vardenafil (Levitra) is not recommended. Beta blockers should not be given to patients with marked sinus bradycardia, greater than first-degree AV block or sick sinus syndrome without a functioning pacemaker, or severe decompensated heart failure, and they should be used with caution in patients with significant bronchospasm, peripheral vascular disease, or diabetes with severe hypoglycemic episodes.

Table 8.1. Results of the Glycemic Effects in Diabetes Mellitus: Carvedilol-Metoprolol Comparison in Hypertensives (GEMINI) Trial

Parameter (Results at 35 weeks)	Carvedilol (n = 454)	Metoprolol (n = 657)	p-Value
Mean change in HbA1c from baseline	0.02	0.15	0.004*
Insulin sensitivity	- 9.1	- 2.0	0.04†
Progression to microalbuminuria	6.6	11.1	0.03

* P-value for the mean difference between groups with respect to the change in HbA1c from baseline (primary outcome). HbA1c was stabilized with carvedilol but increased with metoprolol.

† Insulin resistance was reduced by carvedilol but increased with metoprolol.

From: JAMA 2004;292:2227-2236.

F. **Calcium Antagonists.** Calcium antagonists block or alter cell membrane calcium flux and are useful agents in diabetic patients who require additional drug therapy to lower blood pressure after an ARB (or ACE inhibitor) and a diuretic. In the SYST-EUR trial, long-acting dihydropyridines reduced fatal and nonfatal cardiac events, including sudden death, by 26% and stroke by 42% at 2 years in older patients with isolated systolic hypertension (Lancet 1997;350:757–64); benefits were especially pronounced in diabetic subjects, with reductions in overall mortality of 55%, cardiovascular mortality of 76%, and stroke of 73% (Lancet 1998;351:1755–62). Three recent hypertension megatrials using amlodipine confirmed the efficacy and safety of calcium antagonists for hypertension. In the Antihypertensive and Lipid Lowering treatment to prevent Heart Attack Trial (ALLHAT), there was no difference in combined fatal coronary heart disease and nonfatal MI (or in the risk of cancer or GI bleeding) at 4.8 years among 33,357 hypertensive patients (36% with diabetes) randomized to amlodipine, lisinopril, or chlorthalidone (JAMA 2002;288:2981–97). In the Valsartan Antihypertensive Long-term Use Evaluation (VALUE), there was no difference in fatal and nonfatal cardiac events at 4.2 years among 15,245 high-risk hypertensive patients (32% with diabetes) randomized to amlodipine or valsartan, and the amlodipine-based regimen was associated with greater reductions in blood pressure at 1 month, 6 months, and 1 year (Lancet 2004;363:2022–31). In the Anglo-Scandinavian Cardiac Outcomes Trial-Blood Pressure Lowering Arm (ASCOT-BPLA), the amlodipine-based regimen (perindopril added as needed) resulted in better blood pressure control, fewer major cardiovascular events, and less new-onset diabetes than the atenolol-based regimen (bendroflumethiazide added as needed) at 5.5 years among 19,257 high-risk hypertensive patients (23% with diabetes) (Lancet 2005;366:895-906). In the Conduit Artery Function Evaluation (CAFE), a substudy of ASCOT, the amlodipine-based regimen resulted in lower (4.3 mmHg) central aortic systolic blood pressure and lower (3.0 mmHg) central aortic pulse pressure than the atenolol-based regimen despite nearly identical brachial blood pressure between the two study groups (Circulation 2006;113:1213-25). Once-daily, fixed-dose combination pills—consisting of a calcium antagonist in combination with an ARB, ACE inhibitor, or diuretic—are available and may improve patient compliance by reducing pill burden. A combination pill consisting of amlodipine and atorvastatin (Caduet) is available for the treatment of hypertension and dyslipidemia. Nondihydropyridines should be avoided in patients with severe LV dysfunction, mild to moderate LV dysfunction receiving beta-blockers, sick sinus syndrome, or high-degree AV block. Because of concerns about edema, dihydropyridines should be avoided or used at low initial doses in patients receiving thiazolidinediones.

G. **Vasodilators.** These drugs enter vascular smooth muscle cells to cause direct vasodilation, in contrast to antihypertensive agents that vasodilate by inhibiting hormonal vasoconstrictor mechanisms (e.g., ACE inhibitors), preventing calcium entry into cells that initiate constriction (e.g., calcium antagonists), or blocking alpha-receptor–mediated vasoconstriction (e.g., alpha-1 blockers). Oral direct vasodilators include hydralazine and minoxidil; intravenous agents include hydralazine, nitroprusside, nitroglycerin, and diazoxide. Hydralazine is used infrequently as an antihypertensive agent, although it may be used in conjunction with isosorbide dinitrate as an alternative to angiotensin II receptor blockers in patients with systolic heart failure who are intolerant of ACE inhibitors. It has also been used to treat the hypertension of eclampsia. Adverse effects include tachycardia, angina, headache, dizziness, fluid retention, nasal congestion, lupus-like syndrome, and hepatitis. Minoxidil has become a mainstay for severe hypertension associated with renal insufficiency. Adverse effects include tachycardia, angina, fluid retention, pericardial effusion, and hirsutism. To be fully effective, these direct vasodilators should generally be administered in combination with diuretics and beta blockers. Nitroprusside and nitroglycerin are used for hypertensive crisis.

Chapter 9

Other Measures to Reduce Atherothrombosis

Antiplatelet Therapy

A. **Overview.** Atherothrombotic vascular disease is a dynamic, progressive process of arterial injury, thrombosis, and repair. The resulting atherosclerotic plaque progresses through phases leading to progressive stenosis or acute plaque rupture and intravascular thrombosis, the common underlying mechanism of ischemic stroke, unstable angina, and acute MI (Figure 9.1). Platelet adhesion, activation, and aggregation are central to arterial thrombosis, and antiplatelet therapy has been shown to reduce ischemic stroke, nonfatal MI, and vascular death by 25% in high-risk patients (BMJ 2002;324:71-86). Type 2 diabetic subjects have hyperactive platelets that aggregate more readily in response to platelet agonists, greatly increasing the risk of arterial thrombosis and vascular events.

B. **Aspirin.** Aspirin exerts its antiplatelet effects by blocking the formation of thromboxane A_2 through irreversible acetylation of platelet cyclooxygenase (Figure 9.2). Enzyme inhibition lasts for the lifespan of the platelet (~ 10 days). Aspirin does not prevent atherosclerosis, platelet adhesion, or platelet aggregation in response to ADP, collagen, thrombin, or epinephrine. The Antithrombotic Trialists' Collaborative (ATC) overview of randomized trials of antiplatelet therapy, comprising more than 210,000 patients in 287 studies, found that aspirin reduced the risk of vascular events in high-risk patients by 22% (BMJ 2002;324:71-86). It was estimated that when aspirin is used for secondary prevention, 38 $\pm$ 12 vascular events would be prevented per 1000 diabetic patients. In the Early Treatment Diabetic Retinopathy Study (ETDRS), aspirin (650 mg/d) reduced the risk of MI at 5 years by 26% (9.1% vs. 12.3% for placebo, $p = 0.04$) (JAMA 1992;268:1292-1300). There was no increase

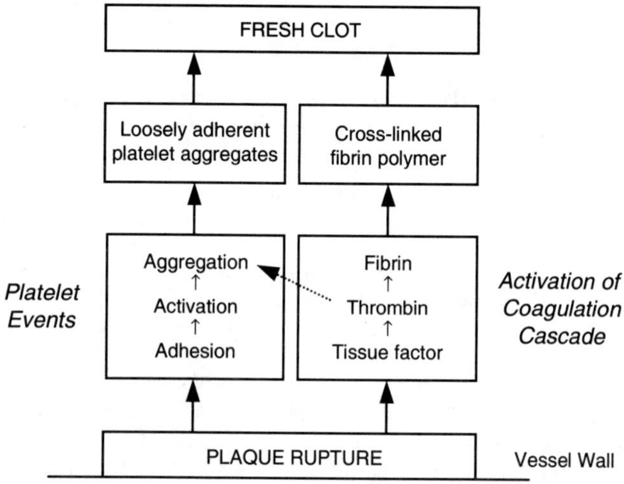

Figure 9.1. Pathophysiology of Atherothrombotic Vascular Disease

Intravascular thrombosis is central to the pathogenesis of acute coronary syndromes and acute ischemic stroke. Plaque rupture exposes circulating blood to vessel wall contents, which rapidly induces clot formation via activation of two complementary systems: platelets and the coagulation cascade. The mechanism of action of antiplatelet agents is shown in Figure 9.2.

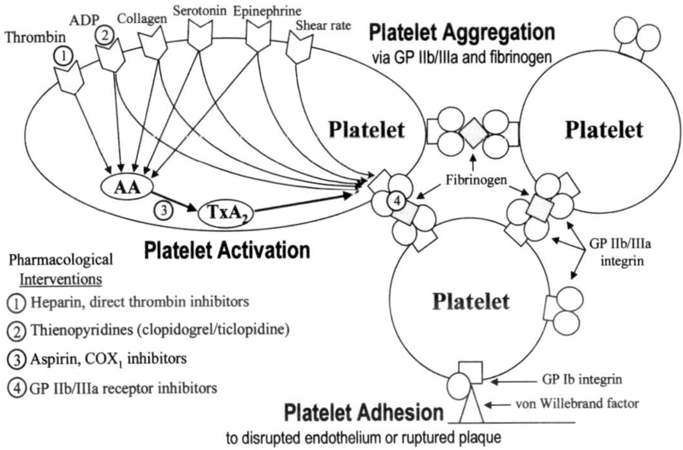

Figure 9.2. Mechanism of Antiplatelet Therapy

AA = arachidonic acid, ADP = adenosine diphosphate, COX = cyclooxygenase, GP = glycoprotein, TXA_2 = thromboxane A_2. Plaque rupture induces platelets to proceed through adhesion, activation, and aggregation. Platelet adhesion is initiated by the binding of von Willebrand factor (vWF), an adhesive glycoprotein released from the injured vessel wall, to the platelet glycoprotein (GP) Ib receptor. Platelets are exposed to multiple agonists at the same time (ADP, TXA_2, epinephrine, thrombin, serotonin, collagen), which trigger a series of events within the platelet, including increased cytosolic calcium, cell shape changes, phosphorylation of proteins, release of granules and lysosomes, arachidonic acid metabolism, and conformational change in the GP IIb/IIIa receptor complex so that it becomes expressed and active on the platelet surface. 50,000-80,000 GP IIb/IIIa receptors reside on the surface of activated platelets. Fibrinogen is the most important ligand of the GP IIb/IIIa receptor and can bind two GP IIa/IIIb receptors simultaneously, creating a molecular platelet-to-platelet bridge. Aspirin blocks the formation of thromboxane A_2 through irreversible acetylation of platelet cyclooxygenase. Clopidogrel and ticlopidine irreversibly modify the platelet ADP receptor, interfering with binding of ADP to its receptor and ADP-mediated activation of the GP IIb/IIIa receptor. Dipyridamole is a phosphodiesterase inhibitor that raises platelet levels of cyclic AMP. Adapted from: Peterson M, Dangas G, Fuster V, in: *The Manual of Interventional Cardiology, 3rd ed.*, Physicians' Press, Royal Oak, MI.

in vitreous or retinal hemorrhage in diabetic patients with established retinopathy receiving aspirin in this study. In the Hypertension Optimal Treatment (HOT) study, aspirin (75 mg/d) reduced the risk of major cardiovascular events (MI, stroke, or cardiovascular death) by 15% and MI by 36% in hypertensive diabetic patients (Lancet 1998;351:1755-62). Among diabetic physicians in the US Physicians Health Study, a primary prevention trial, low-dose aspirin (325 mg every other day) reduced the risk of MI by 61% (4% vs. 10.1% for placebo). These data establish the important role of aspirin for primary and secondary prevention of cardiovascular events in diabetic patients. Recommendations from the American Diabetes Association regarding the use of aspirin are shown in Table 9.1. The optimal dose of aspirin is not known, although ATC found that doses of 75-150 mg/d seem to be as effective as higher doses for long-term therapy. Doses in excess of 325 mg/d are associated with increased risk of gastrointestinal bleeding in a dose-dependent fashion. Low-dose aspirin (75-81 mg/d) should be considered for patients with a history of serious bleeding, especially from the gastrointestinal tract. Many patients with coronary artery disease, prior stroke, or type 2 diabetes are aspirin-resistant (Circulation 2000;18:II-418; Thromb Haemost 2002;88:711-5), which may increase the risk of recurrent vascular events (Circulation 2002;105:1650-5; Thromb Res 1993;71:397-403).

C. **Clopidogrel.** Clopidogrel is an inhibitor of ADP-induced platelet activation and subsequent aggregation, acting by irreversible binding to the platelet $P2Y_{12}$ receptor and of the subsequent ADP-mediated activation of the platelet GP IIb/IIIa receptor complex. Clopidogrel irreversibly modifies the platelet ADP receptor so that platelets exposed to clopidogrel are affected for the remainder of their lifespan. Compared to ticlopidine, another thienopyridine derivative, clopidogrel has a longer duration of action, faster onset of action, and is better tolerated due to fewer gastrointestinal symptoms and adverse hematologic effects (Thromb Haemost 1996;76:939-43; Platelets 1993;4:252-61). In the Clopidogrel vs. Aspirin in Patients at Risk for Ischemic Events (CAPRIE) trial, 19,185 patients with atherosclerotic vascular disease (MI within 35 days, ischemic stroke within 6 months, or established peripheral arterial disease) were randomized to clopidogrel (75 mg/d) or

Table 9.1. Aspirin Therapy in Diabetes: Recommendations from the America Diabetes Association

1. Use aspirin therapy as a secondary prevention strategy in diabetic men and women with evidence of atherosclerotic vascular disease (history of myocardial infarction, vascular bypass procedure, stroke or transient ischemic attack, peripheral vascular disease, claudication, or angina).
2. Consider aspirin therapy as a primary prevention strategy in high-risk men and women with type 1 or type 2 diabetes, including those with:
   - A family history of coronary heart disease
   - Cigarette smoking
   - Hypertension
   - Obesity (>120% desirable weight); BM1 >27.3 kg/m^2 in women or >27.8 kg/m^2 in men
   - Albuminuria (micro or macro)
   - Dyslipidemia: total cholesterol > 200 mg/dL; LDL cholesterol $\geq$ 100 mg/dL; HDL cholesterol < 45 mg/dL in men and < 55 mg/dL in women; triglycerides >200 mg/dL
   - Age > 30 years (use of aspirin has not been studied in younger diabetic subjects)
3. Use enteric-coated aspirin in doses of 81–325 mg/d.
4. People with aspirin allergy, bleeding tendency, anticoagulant therapy, recent gastrointestinal bleeding, and clinically active hepatic disease are not ideal candidates for aspirin therapy. The risks and benefits of aspirin must be carefully considered in these individuals; if aspirin is utilized, the dose should be kept low (81 mg daily).
5. Aspirin therapy should not be recommended for patients under the age of 21 years because of the increased risk of Reye's syndrome associated with aspirin use in this population.

Adapted from: Standards of Medical Care in Diabetes, the American Diabetes Association. Diabetes Care 2007;30(Suppl 1):S4-S41.

aspirin (325 mg/d). At a mean follow-up of 1.9 years, clopidogrel was more effective than aspirin at reducing the combined endpoint of stroke, MI, or vascular death (relative risk reduction 8.7%; p = 0.043) (Lancet 1996;348:1329). Among 3866 patients with type 2 diabetes in CAPRIE, the absolute risk reduction for the primary endpoint was 2.1%, which was larger than the 0.9% reduction seen in a group without diabetes (Am J Cardiol 2002;90:625-8). Clopidogrel resulted in slightly fewer bleeding complications, and there was no difference in the incidence of severe neutropenia between groups. Clopidogrel is approved for the reduction of atherothrombotic events (MI, ischemic stroke, vascular death) in patients with recent MI, recent stroke, or established peripheral arterial disease, and is an excellent choice for high-risk diabetics who require antiplatelet therapy, particularly those intolerant of or allergic to aspirin or who have a cardiovascular event while taking aspirin. The safety profile of clopidogrel is similar to aspirin and better than ticlopidine, with a rare incidence (~ 4 per million) of thrombotic thrombocytopenic purpura (N Engl J Med 2000;342:1773-7).

D. **Combination Aspirin Plus Clopidogrel.** Ex-vivo platelet aggregation studies and recent clinical trials have shown that utilizing two antiplatelet agents with different mechanisms of action is more effective at preventing platelet aggregation and vascular events than single-agent therapy. This was also shown in several clinical trials, including the Clopidogrel in Unstable angina to prevent Recurrent Events (CURE) trial (N Engl J Med 2001;345:494-502); the Clopidogrel as Adjunctive Reperfusion Therapy (CLARITY)-TIMI 28 study (ST-elevation MI < 12 hours treated with fibrinolytic therapy [N Engl J Med 2005;352:1179-89]); the Clopidogrel and Metoprolol in Myocardial Infarction Trial (COMMIT) (acute MI < 24 hours not undergoing primary PCI [Lancet 2005;366:1622-1632]); and the Clopidogrel for the Reduction of Events During Observation (CREDO) trial (elective PCI [JAMA 2002;288:2411-20]). In contrast, no benefit was observed for combination aspirin plus clopidogrel in the Management of ATherothrombosis with Clopidogrel in High-risk patients (MATCH) trial (recent TIA or ischemic stroke at high risk for recurrent ischemic events [Lancet 2004;364:331-337]) or the Clopidogrel for High Atherothrombotic Risk and Ischemic Stabilization Management and Avoidance (CHARISMA) trial (stable vascular disease or multiple risk factors [New Engl J Med 2006;354:1706-17]).

E. **Glycoprotein IIb/IIIa Inhibitors.** GP IIb/IIIa receptor antagonists are the most potent platelet inhibitors available. They exert their antiplatelet effects by blocking the binding of fibrinogen to the GP IIb/IIIa receptor on the platelet surface, the final common pathway of platelet aggregation. GP IIb/IIIa inhibitors block platelet aggregation in response to all platelet agonists (e.g., collagen, thrombin, ADP, epinephrine, thromboxane A_2). Abciximab is a monoclonal antibody and noncompetitive inhibitor that binds 1:1 to the GP IIb/IIIa receptor molecule to induce a conformational change that renders the fibrinogen-binding site of the receptor inactive. Eptifibatide and tirofiban are small-molecule competitive inhibitors of the RGD tripeptide-binding domain of the GP IIb/IIIa receptor. In a pooled analysis of 6458 diabetic subjects enrolled into one of six randomized trials of GP IIb/IIIa inhibitors vs. placebo for medical management of non-ST-elevation acute coronary syndromes (PURSUIT, PRISM, PRISM-PLUS, GUSTO-V, PARAGON A, PARAGON B), GP IIb/IIIa inhibitors reduced 30-day mortality by 26% (4.6% vs. 6.2%, p = 0.007). In a pooled analysis of 1462 diabetic subjects enrolled into one of three randomized trials of GP IIb/IIIa inhibitors vs. placebo as adjuncts to percutaneous coronary intervention (EPIC, EPILOG, EPISTENT), abciximab reduced 1-year mortality by 44% (2.5% vs. 4.5%, p = 0.031) (S. Marso, personal communication). Ongoing trials will help determine the optimal GP IIb/IIIa inhibitor for non-ST-elevation ACS and elective PCI and the role for adjunctive antithrombin therapy (unfractionated heparin, low-molecular-weight heparin, direct thrombin inhibitors) and other antiplatelet agents (aspirin, clopidogrel).

ACE Inhibitors

Angiotensin converting enzyme (ACE) inhibitors block the conversion of angiotensin I to angiotensin II and inhibit the breakdown of bradykinin, resulting in physiologic benefits that confer unique cardioprotective and renoprotective properties to this class of drugs. ACE inhibitors have been shown to improve prognosis following coronary revascularization procedures and in a wide variety of cardiovascular disorders, including hypertension, heart failure, asymptomatic LV dysfunction, MI, proteinuric nephropathy, and diabetic nephropathy/retinopathy/neuropathy. Compelling data from the HOPE and EUROPA trials demonstrate an important role for ACE inhibitors in the prevention of atherothrombotic vascular disease and its complications.

A. **HOPE Study.** The Heart Outcomes Prevention Evaluation (HOPE) study randomized 9297 patients ≥ 55 years with either atherosclerotic arterial disease (prior MI, prior stroke, or peripheral arterial disease) or diabetes plus one additional risk factor (hypertension, elevated total cholesterol, depressed HDL cholesterol, smoking, or microalbuminuria) to ramipril (10 mg/d) or placebo. At a mean follow-up of 5 years, ramipril reduced the primary composite endpoint of MI, stroke, or death from cardiovascular disease by 22% (14.0% vs. 17.8%, $p < 0.001$) (N Engl J Med 2000;342:145-53). In addition, death from cardiovascular causes was reduced by 26% (6.1% vs. 8.1%) and all-cause mortality was reduced by 16% (10.4% vs. 12.2%). Significant risk reduction was also noted for MI (20%), stroke (32%), cardiac arrest (38%), revascularization procedures (15%), and patient-reported new-onset diabetes mellitus (34%). (Ramipril did not reduce new-onset diabetes in DREAM.) The beneficial effects of ramipril were observed in patients with and without diabetes, hypertension, or cardiovascular disease and were independent of the effects of concomitant cardiovascular medications (aspirin, beta-blockers, lipid-lowering agents, other blood pressure drugs). Among 3577 diabetics enrolled in HOPE, ramipril reduced the risk of MI, stroke, or cardiovascular death at 4.5 years by 25% compared to placebo ($p = 0.0004$). Significant risk reduction was noted for death (6.2% vs. 9.7%, $p < 0.001$), MI (10.2% vs. 12.9%, $p = 0.01$), stroke (4.2% vs. 6.1%, $p = 0.007$), and overt nephropathy (6.5% vs. 8.4%, $p = 0.027$) (Lancet 2000;35:253-9). Ramipril is approved to reduce the risk of MI, stroke, and death from cardiovascular causes in patients 55 years or older at high risk of developing a major cardiovascular event because of a history of coronary artery disease, stroke, peripheral arterial disease, or diabetes that is accompanied by at least one other cardiovascular risk factor (hypertension, elevated total cholesterol levels, low HDL levels, cigarette smoking, or documented microalbuminuria). The recommended starting dose is 2.5 mg once daily for 1 week, followed by 5 mg once daily for the next 3 weeks, then increased as tolerated to a maintenance dose of 10 mg once a day (which may be given in 2 divided doses for patients with hypertension or recent MI).

B. **EUROPA and PEACE Trials.** The European Trial with Perindopril in Stable Coronary Artery Disease (EUROPA) was undertaken to evaluate the role of ACE inhibitors on cardiovascular risk in low-risk patients ≥ 18 years without clinical heart failure and with stable coronary heart disease (prior MI > 3 months or coronary revascularization > 6 months before screening, ≥ 70% coronary artery stenosis on angiography, or men with a history of chest pain and a positive stress test). 12% of patients had diabetes (vs. 38% in HOPE), 27% had hypertension (vs. 47% in HOPE), 81% had no angina (vs. 20% in HOPE), and 17% had mild angina. 12,218 men and women were randomized to perindopril 8 mg/d (after tolerating 4 mg/d x 2 weeks) or placebo; half the usual dose was given to patients > 70 years of age. At a mean follow-up of 4.2 years, perindopril reduced the primary composite endpoint of cardiovascular death, MI, or cardiac arrest by 20% (8.0% vs. 9.9%, $p < 0.0003$) (Lancet 2003;362:782-8). The beneficial effects of perindopril were observed in all age groups (≤ 55 years, 56-65 years, > 65 years) and in patients with and without diabetes, hypertension, or prior MI. Benefits were independent of the effects of concomitant cardiovascular medications (aspirin, beta-blockers, lipid-lowering agents, blood pressure drugs). In the Prevention of Events with Angiotensin Converting Enzyme Inhibitors (PEACE) trial, lower-risk patients (compared to HOPE and EUROPA) with stable coronary artery disease and normal/near normal left ventricular function being treated aggressively with coronary revascularization and risk factor modification derived no benefit from the addition of trandolapril at 4.8 years (N Engl J Med 2004;351:2058-68). In this trial, average baseline ejection fraction was 58%, creatinine and cholesterol levels were normal, BP was 133/78 mmHg, and the annualized death rate was only 1.6%, similar to age/sex-matched general population.

C. **Recommendations.** ACE inhibitors are generally safe, well-tolerated, and affordable. Diabetic patients with hypertension, atherosclerotic vascular disease or age ≥ 55 years with at least one other cardiovascular risk factor (hypertension, elevated total cholesterol, low HDL cholesterol, cigarette smoking, microalbuminuria) should be considered for ACE inhibitor therapy. A recent observational study suggests that ACE inhibitors reduce all-cause and cardiovascular-related mortality by 25-50%, even in diabetic patients without cardiovascular disease

(Diabetes Care 2004;27:1330-34). For patients with hypertension or proteinuria or intolerance to ACE inhibitors, an ARB can be used as an alternative. Potential mechanisms for improved cardiovascular prognosis with ACE inhibitors include reductions in left ventricular hypertrophy and arterial wall stress (JAMA 1996;275:1507-13), blood pressure lowering, and improved endothelial function (J Am Coll Cardiol 2000;35:60-6).

Fish Oil

In the GISSI Prevention Study of 11,324 patients with prior MI, 1 gm/d (850 mg of DHA and EPA) of fish oil, a dose too low to affect lipid levels, reduced total mortality by 20% at 3.5 years, including a 45% reduction in sudden cardiac death (Lancet 1999;354:447-55). Similar benefits were seen in DART, in which men with prior MI who were instructed to eat fatty fish at least twice weekly or take a fish oil supplement had a 29% reduction in total mortality (Lancet 1989;2:757-61). In the JELIS trial, 18,600 adults with hypercholesterolemia were randomized to statin alone or statin plus EPA 2 gm/d. The statin plus EPA group experienced a 19% reduction ($p = 0.01$) in major adverse coronary events at 5 years (American Heart Association meeting, November, 2005, Dallas, Texas). Consumption of fish and omega-3 fatty acids has also been shown to reduce the risk of CHD in otherwise healthy persons and is an important component of the Mediterranean-style diet (Chapter 4). Individuals with diabetes should be instructed to eat at least 2 servings of fish high in omega-3 fats per week. High-dose fish oil supplements (3-10 gm/d) can be used to lower triglyceride levels (Chapter 7). Omacor, which contains highly purified omega-3 or acid ethyl esters, mainly EPA and DHA, has been approved by the FDA for the treatment of triglyceride levels ≥ 500 mg/dL. In clinical studies, the daily dose was 4 gm/day.

Alcohol

Most observational studies show that people who consume 2-14 drinks per week (ideally 1 drink per day or every other day) have lower rates of cardiovascular events and all-cause mortality compared to nondrinkers. The benefits of moderate alcohol intake are even more impressive in diabetic individuals compared to the general population. One drink is defined as 12 ounces of beer, 5.5 ounces of wine, or 1.5 ounces of 80-proof distilled liquor (spirits). However, blood pressure and triglycerides rise proportionately with alcohol intake of more than 3 drinks per day; at this level of alcohol consumption, the reduction in cardiovascular mortality is offset by the increased risk of cancer, strokes, and accidents. Optimal intake of alcohol is not more than 2 drinks daily for men or 1 drink daily for women. Although moderate alcohol consumption (up to 1 oz ethanol per day) has been associated with a lower risk of CHD, it is not recommended as a therapeutic agent because of possible deleterious effects, such as hypertriglyceridemia, hypertension and increased risk of breast and other cancers, and because of the risk for abuse with larger intakes.

Influenza and Pneumococcal Vaccination

Influenza epidemics occur most often during the winter months and are responsible for more than 40,000 deaths each year in the U.S. alone. To prevent hospitalization and death, the Advisory Committee on Immunization Practices (ACIP) recommends annual influenza vaccination for higher-risk individuals, including those with type 2 diabetes (www.cdc.gov). Patients with type 2 diabetes should also receive Pneumovax to reduce the risk for pneumococcal pneumonia (primary dose: 0.5 mL; one-time booster at 5 years if primary dose is received before age 65).

Chapter 10. Clinical Trials

Table 10.1. Diabetes Care Trials

Trial	Design	Results
ADOPT: A Diabetes Outcome Progression Trial (N Engl J Med 2006;355:2427-43)	4,360 treatment-naive patients with type 2 diabetes were randomized to 4 years of treatment with rosiglitazone, metformin, or glyburide. Primary outcome: time to monotherapy failure (FPG > 180 mg/dL).	Cumulative incidence of monotherapy failure at 5 years was significantly less for rosiglitazone (15%) compared to either metformin (21%) or glyburide (34%), representing risk reductions of 32% and 63%, respectively ($p < 0.001$ for both comparisons).
DCCT: Diabetes Control and Complications Trial (N Engl J Med 2005;353:2643-2653)	1,441 patients aged 13-39 years with type 1 diabetes were randomized to intensive blood glucose control vs. normal care. Follow-up: 20 years.	Intensive glucose control reduced the combined endpoint of major macrovascular events by 50% ($p = 0.082$). MI was 5 times more frequent with conventional treatment (0.29 vs. 0.06 events/100 patients years, $p = 0.065$).
DIGAMI: Diabetes Mellitus Insulin Glucose Infusion in Acute Myocardial Infarction (J Am Coll Cardiol 1995;26:57-65)	620 patients with diabetes and acute MI were randomized to insulin and glucose infusion (followed by SQ insulin post-discharge for 3 months) vs. conventional therapy.	Insulin treatment was associated with a 29% decrease in mortality at 1 year ($p = 0.027$).

See p. 1 for abbreviations

Table 10.1. Diabetes Care Trials

Trial	Design	Results
DPP: Diabetes Prevention Project (N Engl J Med 2002;346:393-403)	3,234 patients with elevated fasting and post-load glucose levels (but not diabetes) were randomized to lifestyle intervention (≥ 150 minutes of exercise/week and a weight-loss diet), metformin (850 mg bid), or placebo.	Lifestyle modification decreased the incidence of new diabetes by 58% ($p < 0.001$ vs. placebo), and metformin decreased the incidence of new diabetes by 31% ($p < 0.001$ vs. placebo) over 2.8 years of follow-up.
DREAM: Diabetes Reduction Assessment with Ramipril and Rosiglitazone Medication (Lancet 2006;368:1096-1105)	5,269 patients aged ≥ 30 years with IFG (mean FPG 104 mg/dL) or IGT (mean 2-hour post-challenge blood glucose 156 mg/dL) were randomized to rosiglitazone 8 mg/d or placebo in a factorial design. Primary endpoint: new diabetes or death. Follow-up: 3 years.	Rosiglitazone reduced the primary endpoint by 60% (11.6% vs. 26.0%, $p < 0.0001$). Additionally, reversion to normoglycemia occurred more often with rosiglitazone (50.5% vs. 30.3% for placebo, $p < 0.0001$). Cardiovascular event rates were similar, except for CHF (0.5% for rosiglitazone vs. 0.1% for placebo, $p = 0.01$).
Expert Committee on the Diagnosis and Classification of Diabetes Mellitus (Diabetes Care 2003;26:3160-7)	An international expert committee was convened to reexamine 1997 classification and diagnostic criteria for diabetes mellitus.	Fasting plasma glucose (FPG) level diagnostic of impaired fasting glucose (prediabetes) was lowered from 110 mg/dL to 100 mg/dL. This redefines normal FPG as < 100 mg/dL.
Finnish Diabetes Prevention Study (N Engl J Med 2001;344:1343-1350)	522 overweight men and women (mean age 55 years) were randomized to a control group or intensive counseling for weight control, saturated fat intake, fiber intake, and physical activity. Mean follow-up: 3.2 years.	Intensive counseling and lifestyle modification led to a 58% decrease in the risk of developing new diabetes (11% vs. 23%, $p < 0.001$). Amount of weight loss was greater in the intervention group (3.5 kg vs. 0.8 kg, $p < 0.001$).

See p. 1 for abbreviations

Table 10.1. Diabetes Care Trials

Trial	Design	Results
Gomez-Perez et al. Efficacy and Safety of Rosiglitazone plus Metformin in Mexicans with Type 2 Diabetes (Diabetes Metab Res Rev 2002;18:127-134)	116 Mexican patients with diabetes and poor glucose control on metformin alone were randomized to rosiglitazone 2 or 4 mg bid or placebo in addition to metformin 2.5 g/d. Follow-up: 24 weeks.	HbA_{1c} decreased with rosiglitazone therapy in addition to metformin (2 mg bid: –0.7%, $p = 0.005$; 4 mg bid: –1.2%, $p < 0.001$). It was unchanged in the placebo group. Mean fasting glucose also decreased with rosiglitazone ($p < 0.002$). Total-to-HDL ratio remained unchanged.
Indian Diabetes Prevention Program (Diabetologia 2006;49:289-97)	421 men and 110 women with IGT were randomized to a control group, a lifestyle modification group, a metformin group, or a metformin plus lifestyle modification group x 30 months.	Compared to control, the risk of new-onset diabetes was reduced by lifestyle modification (28.5% reduction, $p = 0.018$), metformin (26.4% reduction, $p = 0.029$), and lifestyle modification plus metformin (28.2% reduction, $p = 0.022$).
MRFIT: Multiple Risk Factor Intervention Trial (Diabetes Care 1993;16:435-444)	347,978 men (5,163 taking medication for diabetes) were enrolled and followed for a mean of 12 years to compare the risk of CV death in men with and without diabetes and to assess predictors of CV mortality.	There were 160 deaths per 10,000 person-years in the diabetes group compared with 53.2 in the non-diabetic group. After adjusting for age, race, cholesterol, BP and smoking, mortality remained three times greater in men with diabetes.

See p. 1 for abbreviations

Table 10.1. Diabetes Care Trials

Trial	Design	Results
Steno-2 Study (N Engl J Med 2003;348:383-393)	160 diabetic patients with microalbuminuria (mean age 55.1 years) were randomized to conventional treatment to national guidelines or to intensive treatment (behavior modification; medical therapy for hyperglycemia, hypertension, dyslipidemia, and microalbuminuria; and aspirin). Follow-up: 7.8 years.	Intensive therapy led to significant reductions in CV disease (53%), nephropathy (61%), retinopathy (58%), and autonomic neuropathy (63%). There were significant reductions in HbA_{1c}, BP, total cholesterol, triglycerides, and urinary albumin excretion rate.
STOP-NIDDM: Study to Prevent NIDDM (Lancet 2002;359:2072-2077)	1,429 patients with impaired glucose tolerance were randomized to acarbose 100 mg tid or placebo. Follow-up: 3.9 years.	Acarbose reduced the risk of new diabetes by 25% ($p = 0.0015$), new hypertension by 24% ($p = 0.0059$), and CV events by 40% ($p = 0.027$).
TRIPOD: Troglitazone in the Prevention of Diabetes (Diabetes 2002;51:2796-2803)	266 Hispanic women with a history of gestational diabetes were randomized to troglitazone 400 mg/d or placebo. Follow-up: 2.5 years.	Troglitazone reduced the incidence of new diabetes by 56% ($p < 0.01$) and maintained lower incidence off drug for 10 months
UKPDS 33: United Kingdom Prospective Diabetes Study (Lancet 1998;352: 837-853)	3,867 men and women with newly diagnosed diabetes were randomized to intensive blood glucose control (insulin or a sulfonylurea) or conventional care (diet modification). Follow-up: 10 years.	HbA_{1c} was 11% lower in the intensive care group (7.0% vs. 7.9%). This was associated with a 12% lower risk for any diabetes-related endpoint ($p = 0.029$) and non-significant reductions in diabetes-related death (10%, $p = 0.34$) and all-cause mortality (6%, $p = 0.44$).

See p. 1 for abbreviations

Table 10.1. Diabetes Care Trials

Trial	Design	Results
UKPDS 34: United Kingdom Prospective Diabetes Study (Lancet 1998;352: 854-865)	753 men and women with newly diagnosed diabetes and obesity (> 120% ideal body weight) were randomized to intensive blood glucose control with metformin or conventional care (diet modification). Follow-up: 10.7 years.	Metformin reduced the risk of diabetes-related complications by 32% ($p = 0.002$), diabetes-related death by 42% ($p = 0.017$), and all-cause mortality by 36% ($p = 0.11$). Secondary analysis showed metformin was more effective in reducing endpoints than sulfonylureas or insulin.
UKPDS 35: United Kingdom Prospective Diabetes Study (BMJ 2000;321: 405-412)	4,585 men and women with diabetes were randomized to intensive blood glucose control (insulin or a sulfonylurea) or conventional care (diet modification). Follow-up: 10 years.	Each 1% decrease in HbA_{1c} reduced the risk of diabetes-related complications by 21% ($p < 0.0001$), diabetes-related death by 21% ($p < 0.0001$), MI by 14% ($p < 0.0001$), and microvascular complications by 37% ($p < 0.0001$). No threshold of risk was observed for any endpoint.
XENDOS: Xenical in the Prevention of Diabetes in Obese Subjects (Rev Med Liege 2002;57:617-621)	3,304 obese patients (BMI ≥ 30 kg/m^2 were randomized to orlistat or lifestyle modification for weight loss and to evaluate its effect on the incidence of diabetes. Follow-up: 4 years.	Orlistat treatment led to a 37% relative reduction in new diabetes (6.2% vs. 9.0%, $p = 0.003$). The group with impaired glucose tolerance and weight loss had a greater absolute reduction (19% vs. 29%, $p < 0.005$).

See p. 1 for abbreviations

Table 10.2. Diabetes Epidemiology Studies

Trial	Design	Results
ARIC: Atherosclerosis Risk in Communities Study (Ann Intern Med 2000;81-91)	1,676 patients aged 45-64 with diabetes and no known CHD were followed for 8 years to examine the association of traditional and nontraditional CHD risk factors in patients with diabetes.	186 (11.1%) developed CHD, and risk was related to traditional risk factors (high LDL, low HDL, hypertension, smoking). Markers of inflammation (low albumin, high fibrinogen, high von Willebrand factor, high leukocyte count) also correlated with development of CHD.
DECODE: Diabetes Epidemiology Collaborative Analysis of Diagnostic Criteria in Europe (Lancet 1999;354:617-621)	Over 25,000 patients from 13 European trials were analyzed to compare the mortality of patients meeting ADA criteria for diabetes (fasting plasma glucose > 126 mg/dL only) with those meeting the WHO criteria (2-hour post-load glucose > 200 mg/dL).	Using ADA criteria, the hazard ratio for death was 1.81 for men and 1.79 for women (vs. normal glucose tolerance). For those meeting WHO criteria, the hazard ratio for death was 2.02 in men and 2.77 in women. Those with normal fasting glucose and impaired 2-hour glucose tolerance had the greatest risk of death.
Norhammer et al. Glucose Metabolism in Patients with Acute MI and no Previous Diagnosis of Diabetes Mellitus (Lancet 2002;359: 2140- 2144)	181 consecutive patients (mean age 63.5 years) who were admitted with acute MI, no known DM, and glucose < 200 mg/dL were given a standard oral glucose tolerance test at discharge and 3 months to define the prevalence of impaired glucose tolerance (IGT).	At hospital discharge, 35% of patients had IGT, and 31% had unrecognized diabetes. At 3 months, 40% had IGT and 25% were diagnosed with diabetes.

See p. 1 for abbreviations

Table 10.2. Diabetes Epidemiology Studies

Trial	Design	Results
Nurses' Health Study (N Engl J Med 2001;345:790-797, Am J Public Health 2000;90:1490-1415)	84,941 women aged 38-63 years with no history of diabetes or CHD were followed for 10 years to identify factors predisposing to the development of diabetes.	91% of diabetes (n = 3,300) could be attributed to habits and forms of behavior that did not conform to the low-risk pattern (diet rich in whole grains and low in trans-fats and glycemic load, exercise, abstinence from smoking, and ≥ ½ alcoholic beverage daily). Women in the low-risk group had a relative risk of diabetes of 0.09 (95% CI, 0.05 to 0.17).
Physician's Health Study (JAMA 1992;268:63-67)	21,271 male US physicians aged 40-84 years were enrolled and followed for 5 years to assess the effect of vigorous exercise on the development of diabetes.	Those who exercised at least once weekly had a 37% lower incidence of new diabetes than those who exercised less often ($p < 0.001$).
Physician's Health Study – Diabetic Subgroup (Arch Intern Med 2001;161:242-247)	2,317 male US physicians with diabetes and 815 with both diabetes and CHD aged 40-84 years were enrolled and followed for 5 years to assess the impact of diabetes on all-cause and CHD mortality.	The relative risk for all-cause mortality was 2.3 for men with diabetes and 4.7 for men with diabetes and CHD. The relative risk for CHD death was 3.3 with diabetes, and 12.0 for those with both diabetes and CHD.
Sinha et al. Prevalence of Impaired Glucose Tolerance among Children and Adolescents with Marked Obesity (N Engl J Med 2002:346:820-810)	55 children (aged 4-10 years) and 112 adolescents (aged 11-18 years) with a body mass index greater than the 95th percentile for age and sex underwent 2-hour oral glucose tolerance testing.	Impaired glucose tolerance (fasting plasma glucose < 126 mg/dL and 2-hour plasma glucose 140-200 mg/dL) was detected in 25% of obese children and 22% of obese adolescents.

See p. 1 for abbreviations

Chapter 11

Diabetes Drug Summaries

This section contains prescribing information pertinent to the clinical use of common diabetic medications, as compiled from a variety of sources (see below). The information provided is not exhaustive, and the reader is referred to other drug information references and the manufacturer's product literature for further information. Clinical use of the information provided and any consequences that may arise from its use are the responsibilities of the prescribing physician. The authors, editors, and publisher do not warrant or guarantee the information contained in this section, and do not assume and expressly disclaim any liability for errors or omissions or any consequences that may occur from such. The use of any drug should be preceded by careful review of the package insert, which provides indications and dosing approved by the U.S. Food and Drug Administration. (Package inserts can be found on the websites provided at the end of each drug summary.) Drugs are listed alphabetically by generic name; trade names follow in parentheses. To search by trade name, consult the index. Safety in pregnancy listing is designated by the U.S. Food and Drug Administration's (USFDA) use-in-pregnancy letter code (Table 11.1, next page).

Drug References:

1. American Association of Clinical Endocrinologists and American College of Clinical Endocrinologists. Medical Guidelines for the Management of Diabetes Mellitus: The AACE System of Intensive Diabetes Self-Management – 2002 Update. Endocr Pract 2002;8(Suppl 1).
2. Physician's Desk Reference (PDR), 2006.
3. Drug Facts and Comparisons, 2006.
4. Zangeneh F, Kudva YC, Basu A. Insulin sensitizers. Mayo Clin Proc 2003;78:471-479.
5. DeWitt, DE, Hirsch IB. Outpatient insulin therapy in type 1 diabetes mellitus. JAMA 2003;289:2254-2264.
6. Inzucchi SE. Oral antihyperglycemic therapy for type 2 diabetes. JAMA 2002;287:360-372.
7. Nathan DM. Initial management of glycemia in type 2 diabetes mellitus. N Engl J Med 2002;347:1342-1349.

Table 11.1. USFDA Use-in-Pregnancy Letter Code

Category	Interpretation
A	**Controlled studies show no risk.** Adequate, well-controlled studies in pregnant women have not shown a risk to the fetus in any trimester of pregnancy.
B	**No evidence of risk in humans.** Adequate, well-controlled studies in pregnant women have not shown increased risk of fetal abnormalities despite adverse findings in animals, or, in the absence of adequate human studies, animal studies show no fetal risk. The chance of fetal harm is remote, but remains a possibility.
C	**Risk cannot be ruled out.** Adequate, well-controlled human studies are lacking, and animal studies have shown a risk to the fetus or are lacking. There is a chance of fetal harm if the drug is administered during pregnancy, but potential benefit from use of the drug may outweigh potential risk.
D	**Positive evidence of risk.** Studies in humans or investigational or post-marketing data have demonstrated fetal risk. Nevertheless, potential benefit from use of the drug may outweigh potential risk. For example, the drug may be acceptable if needed in a life-threatening situation or serious disease for which safer drugs cannot be used or are ineffective.
X	**Contraindicated in pregnancy.** Studies in animals or humans or investigational or post-marketing reports have demonstrated positive evidence of fetal abnormalities or risk which clearly outweigh any possible benefit to the patient.

Chapter 11

Diabetes Drug Summaries

Acarbose (Precose)

Class: Alpha-glucosidase inhibitor

Mechanism of Action: These drugs act locally in the small intestine by inhibiting alpha-glucosidase enzymes; this action slows digestion of ingested carbohydrates, delays glucose absorption, and reduces the increase in postprandial blood glucose.

Clinical Effects: Alpha-glucosidase inhibitors cause a 0.5-1% reduction in HbA1c and have no significant effect on fasting blood glucose levels.

Dosage: 25 mg three times/day with the first bite of each main meal. Maintenance dose ranges are 50-100 mg three times/day. Dose adjustments should be made at 4-8 week intervals. Maximum dosage ≤ 60 kg = 50 mg tid; > 60 kg = 100 mg tid.

Renal Impairment: Not recommended in patients with CrCl < 25 mL/min.

Hepatic Impairment: No dosage adjustment necessary.

Contraindications: Major GI disorders, including inflammatory bowel disease, chronic ulceration, malabsorption, or partial intestinal obstruction. Not recommended for use in patients with CrCl < 25 mL/min.

Adverse Effects: Abdominal bloating, flatulence, diarrhea. Adverse GI effects tend to diminish with continued treatment.

Monitoring: HbA1c, FBG, LFT's (every 3 months).

Drug Interactions: Decreased acarbose effect with intestinal adsorbents (charcoal) and digestive enzyme preparations (amylase, pancreatin).

Safety in Pregnancy: B

Comments: Most useful in patients with postprandial hyperglycemia; not associated with hypoglycemia or weight gain. Must use glucose and not complex sugars to reverse hypoglycemia, if it occurs.

Dosage Forms: 25 mg, 50 mg, 100 mg tablets.

Website: www.pdr.net

Exenatide (Byetta)

Class: Incretin mimetic

Mechanism of Action: Incretins, such as glucagon-like peptide-1, enhance glucose-dependent insulin secretion and exhibit other antihyperglycemic actions following their release into the circulation from the gut. Exenatide is an incretin mimetic agent that enhances glucose-dependent insulin secretion by the pancreatic beta-cell, suppresses inappropriately elevated glucagon secretion, and slows gastric emptying.

Clinical Effects: Exenatide, in combination with metformin, a sulfonylurea, or both, reduces HbA1c by 0.4-1.1%, fasting blood glucose by

10-25 mg/dL, 2-hour post-prandial blood glucose by 60-70 mg/dL, and body weight by 0.9-3.6 kg.
Dosage: Starting dose is 5 mcg twice a day, given within the 60-minute period before the morning and evening meals. The dose can be increased to 10 mcg twice daily after 1 month of therapy. Each dose should be administered subcutaneously in the abdomen, thigh, or upper arm. When exenatide is added to metformin therapy, the current dose of metformin can be kept the same. When exenatide is added to sulfonylurea therapy, a reduction in the dose of sulfonylurea may be considered to reduce the risk of hypoglycemia.
Renal Impairment: Not recommended in patients with end-stage renal disease or severe renal impairment (creatinine clearance < 30 mL/min).
Hepatic Impairment: No dosage adjustment necessary.
Contraindications: Type 1 diabetes, end-stage renal disease or severe renal impairment (creatinine clearance < 30 mL/min), severe gastrointestinal disease.
Adverse Effects: Hypoglycemia, nausea, vomiting, diarrhea, feeling jittery, dizziness, headache, dyspepsia.
Monitoring: HbA1c, FBG.
Drug Interactions: The effects of exenatide to slow gastric emptying may reduce the extent and rate of absorption of orally administered drugs, so it should be used with caution in patients receiving oral medications that require rapid gastrointestinal absorption. Medications that are dependent on threshold concentrations for efficacy, such as contraceptives, levothyroxine, and antibiotics, should be taken at least 1 hour before exenatide injection. If such drugs are to be administered with food, they should be taken with a meal or snack when exenatide is not administered.
Safety in Pregnancy: C
Comments: Exenatide is indicated for type 2 diabetic patients who are taking metformin, a sulfonylurea, or both, but have not achieved adequate glycemic control.
Dosage Forms: 5 and 10 mcg pre-filled pen injectors, 60 doses each
Website: www.byetta.com

Glimepiride (Amaryl)

Class: Sulfonylurea
Mechanism of Action: Sulfonylureas stimulate insulin release by blocking the potassium channel of the beta cell. They also decrease hepatic glucose production and may improve insulin sensitivity at the receptor and post-receptor levels.
Clinical Effects: Sulfonylureas reduce HbA1c by up to 1-2% and fasting blood glucose by up to 60-80 mg/dL.
Dosage: Initial dose is 1-2 mg/day. May increase dose at 1-2 week intervals, with usual maintenance doses of 1-4 mg/day. Maximum dose is 8 mg/day. Elderly patients should be started at doses of 1 mg/day.
Renal Impairment: CrCl < 22 mL/min: initial dosage = 1 mg.
Hepatic Impairment: No data available.

Contraindications: Hypersensitivity, type 1 diabetes, diabetic ketoacidosis.
Adverse Effects: Headache, dizziness, weakness, nausea.
Monitoring: HbA1c, FBG.
Safety in Pregnancy: C
Dosage Forms: 1 mg, 2 mg, 4 mg tablets.
Website: www.amaryl.com

Glipizide (Glucotrol/Glucotrol XL)

Class: Sulfonylurea
Mechanism of Action: Sulfonylureas stimulate insulin release by blocking the potassium channel of the beta cell. They also decrease hepatic glucose production and may improve insulin sensitivity at the receptor and post-receptor levels.
Clinical Effects: Sulfonylureas reduce HbA1c by up to 1-2% and fasting blood glucose by up to 60-80 mg/dL.
Dosage:
Glipizide (Glucotrol) is given at a starting dose of 5 mg, 30 minutes before a meal. Geriatric patients or those with liver disease may be started on 2.5 mg. Maintenance doses range from 2.5 to 40 mg/day; however doses above 20 mg generally do not provide greater blood glucose reduction. Single doses above 15 mg should be divided.
Glipizide-GITS (Glucotrol XL)
Glipizide-GITS is given at a starting dose of 5 mg/day. Maintenance doses range from 5-20 mg/day.
Renal Impairment: No dosage adjustment necessary.
Hepatic Impairment: Initial dosage should be 2.5 mg/day.
Warnings/Contraindications: Sulfonylurea allergy, type 1 diabetes.
Adverse Effects: Headache, anorexia, nausea, vomiting, diarrhea, epigastric fullness, constipation, heartburn, rash, hives, photosensitivity, edema, hypoglycemia.
Drug Interactions: Fluconazole increases levels of glipizide.
Monitoring: HbA1c, FBG.
Safety in Pregnancy: C
Comments: More effective when given 30 minutes before meals. When changing from immediate to sustained release, use same total daily dose.
Dosage Forms: 5 and 10 mg tablet; 5 and 10 mg extended-release tablets.
Website: www.pdr.net

Glipizide/Metformin (Metaglip)

Class: Sulfonylurea/biguanide
Mechanism of Action: Sulfonylureas stimulate insulin release by blocking the potassium channel of the beta cell. They also decrease hepatic glucose production and may improve insulin sensitivity at the receptor and post-receptor levels. Metformin increases insulin sensitivity in the liver by inhibiting hepatic gluconeogenesis and/or glycogenolysis, thereby reducing hepatic glucose production. It also enhances muscle glucose uptake and utilization.
Clinical Effects: When used as initial therapy, Metaglip reduced HbA_{1c} by up

to 2.15% and fasting blood glucose by up to 55 mg/dL.

Dosage:

Initial therapy: 2.5/250 mg once a day with a meal; if FBG is 280-320 mg/dL, start with 2.5/500 mg twice a day with meals; may increase by one tablet per day every two weeks to a maximum of 10/2000 mg per day, given in divided doses.

Second-line therapy: (patients not controlled on a sulfonylurea or metformin alone): Start with 2.5/500 mg or 5/500 mg twice a day with meals; may increase up to a maximum of 20/2000 mg per day, given in divided doses.

Renal Impairment: Do not use in patients with renal insufficiency (serum creatinine ≥ 1.5 mg/dL in men or ≥ 1.4 mg/dL in women).

Hepatic Impairment: Do not use with severe liver disease.

Contraindications: Metformin should not be given to anyone ≥ 80 years of age without first documenting a normal creatinine clearance. Because of the metformin component, do not use in renal insufficiency (serum creatinine ≥ 1.5 mg/dL in men or ≥ 1.4 mg/dL in women), in patients receiving iodinated contrast material (discontinue temporarily for 48 hours after procedure because of potential for acute alteration of renal function, and do not resume until normal renal function has been documented), or in patients prone to metabolic acidosis or hypoxic states (liver failure, congestive heart failure requiring pharmacological therapy, diabetic ketoacidosis, major surgical procedures, sepsis, severe trauma, alcoholism, COPD); these conditions increase the risk of developing lactic acidosis. Not recommended for type 1 diabetes.

Adverse Effects: Anorexia, nausea, abdominal discomfort, diarrhea, metallic taste, vitamin B_{12} deficiency, lactic acidosis, hypoglycemia, headache, dizziness, rash, photosensitivity reactions.

Drug Interactions: Fluconazole increases levels of glipizide; cimetidine increases blood levels of metformin

Monitoring: Renal function, HbA_{1c}, FBG, hematologic parameters (Hb, hematocrit, RBC indices).

Safety in Pregnancy: C

Comments: Give with meals. Patients already on glipizide and metformin may be switched to the nearest equivalent dose of the combination product.

Dosage Forms: 2.5/250 mg, 2.5/500 mg, 5/500 mg tablets.

Website: www.metaglip.com

Glyburide (DiaBeta, Micronase, Glynase)

Class: Sulfonylurea

Mechanism of Action: Sulfonylureas stimulate insulin release by blocking the potassium channel of the beta cell. They also decrease hepatic glucose production and may improve insulin sensitivity at the receptor and post-receptor levels.

Clinical Effects: Sulfonylureas reduce HbA1c by up to 1-2% and fasting blood glucose by up to 60-80 mg/dL.

Dosage: Glyburide (DiaBeta/Micronase) is given at a starting dose of 2.5-5 mg daily; maintenance doses range from 2.5-20 mg/day in 1 or 2 divided doses. Glyburide (Glynase) has a starting dose of 1.5-3 mg daily; maintenance doses range from 3-12 mg/day in 1 or 2 divided doses.
Renal Impairment: CrCl 10-50 mL/min: use conservative initial and maintenance doses. CrCl < 10 mL/min: avoid use.
Hepatic Impairment: Use conservative initial and maintenance doses.
Contraindications: Hypersensitivity, type 1 diabetes.
Adverse Effects: Hypoglycemia, hypersensitivity, weight gain, nausea/abdominal pain. headache, dizziness, rash, photosensitivity reactions.
Monitoring: HbA1c, FBG.
Safety in Pregnancy: C
Comments: Most effective when given 30 minutes before meals.
Dosage Forms: Diabeta: 1.25 mg, 2.5 mg, 5 mg tablets; Glynase: 1.5 mg, 3 mg micronized tablets.
Website: www.pdr.net

Glyburide/Metformin (Glucovance)

Class: Sulfonylurea/biguanide
Mechanism of Action: Sulfonylureas stimulate insulin release by blocking the potassium channel of the beta cell. They also decrease hepatic glucose production and may improve insulin sensitivity at the receptor and post-receptor levels. Metformin increases insulin sensitivity in the liver by inhibiting hepatic gluconeogenesis and thereby reducing hepatic glucose production. It also enhances muscle glucose uptake and utilization.
Clinical Effects: When used as initial therapy in drug-naïve patients, Glucovance reduced HbA_{1c} by up to 1.5% and fasting blood glucose by up to 50 mg/dL.
Dosage:
Initial therapy: 1.25/250 mg once or twice a day with meals. May titrate up to a total daily dose of 10/2000 mg. (Glucovance 5/500 mg should not be used as initial therapy due to risk of hypoglycemia.)
Second-line therapy (patients not adequately controlled on a sulfonylurea or metformin alone): 2.5/500 mg or 5/500 mg twice a day with meals. Maximum recommended daily dose is 20/2000 mg.
Renal Impairment: Do not use in patients with renal insufficiency (serum creatinine ≥ 1.5 mg/dL in men or ≥ 1.4 mg/dL in women).
Hepatic Impairment: Do not use with severe liver disease.
Contraindications: Metformin should not be given to anyone ≥ 80 years of age without first documenting a normal creatinine clearance. Because of the metformin component, do not use in renal insufficiency (serum creatinine ≥ 1.5 mg/dL in men or ≥ 1.4 mg/dL in women), in patients receiving iodinated contrast material (discontinue temporarily for 48 hours after procedure because of potential for acute alteration

renal function, and do not resume until normal renal function has been documented), or in the presence of any condition associated with hypoxemia, dehydration, metabolic acidosis or sepsis (liver failure, binge drinking, congestive heart failure requiring pharmacological therapy, diabetic ketoacidosis, major surgical procedures, sepsis, severe trauma, alcoholism, binge drinking, COPD); these conditions increase the risk of developing lactic acidosis. Not recommended for type 1 diabetes.

Adverse Effects: Anorexia, nausea, abdominal discomfort, diarrhea, metallic taste, vitamin B_{12} deficiency, lactic acidosis, hypoglycemia, weight gain, headache, dizziness, rash, photosensitivity reactions.

Monitoring: Renal function, HbA_{1c}, FBG, hematologic parameters (Hb, hematocrit, RBC indices).

Drug Interactions: Cimetidine increases blood levels of metformin.

Safety in Pregnancy: C

Comments: Give with meals. Patients already on glyburide and metformin may be switched to the nearest equivalent dose of the combination product.

Dosage Forms: 1.25/250 mg, 2.5/500 mg, 5/500 mg tablets.

Website: www.glucovance.com

Inhaled Human Insulin (Exubera)

Class: Rapid-acting insulin

Mechanism of Action: The primary activity of insulin is regulation of glucose metabolism. Insulin lowers blood glucose concentrations by stimulating peripheral glucose uptake by skeletal muscle and fat, and by inhibiting hepatic glucose production. Insulin inhibits lipolysis in the adipocyte, inhibits proteolysis, and enhances protein synthesis.

Dosage: Doses should be administered immediately prior to meals (no more than 10 minutes prior to each meal). A 1-mg blister of Exubera inhaled insulin is approximately equal to 3 units of subcutaneously injected regular human insulin. A 3-mg blister of Exubera is approximately equal to 8 units of subcutaneously injected regular human insulin. (Note that 3 x 1-mg blisters are not equal to 1 x 3-mg blister.) Patients should combine 1 mg and 3 mg blisters so that the least number of blisters per dose are taken. Initial pre-meal doses may be calculated using the following formula: [body weight (kg) x 0.05 mg/kg = pre-meal dose (mg)] rounded down to the nearest whole milligram number (e.g., 3.7 mg rounded down to 3 mg). Approximate guidelines for initial pre-meal Exubera doses are listed in Table 11.3 (p. 174).

Renal Impairment: Dose requirements may be reduced in patients with renal impairment.

Hepatic Impairment: Dose requirements may be reduced in patients with hepatic impairment.

Contraindications: Underlying lung disease (asthma, COPD); patients who smoke or who have discontinued smoking less than 6 months prior to starting therapy. If a patient starts or resumes smoking, Exubera must be discontinued immediately due to the increased risk of hypoglycemia, and an alternative treatment must be utilized.
Adverse Effects: Hypoglycemia, dry mouth, cough, dyspnea, pharyngitis, chest discomfort, decreased pulmonary function.
Monitoring: HbA_{1c}, FBG, pulmonary function tests (prior to initiation, at 6 months, and then annually).
Drug Interactions: Bronchodilators and other inhaled products may alter the absorption of inhaled insulin. Consistent timing of bronchodilator dosing relative to Exubera administration is recommended.
Safety in Pregnancy: C
Comments: Exubera has a more rapid onset of glucose-lowering activity compared to subcutaneously injected regular human insulin but a similar duration of action. In patients with type 2 diabetes, Exubera can be used as monotherapy, or in combination with oral agents or longer-acting insulins. Patients with type 1 diabetes can use Exubera also, but will need to include a longer-acting insulin in their regimen. The inhaler must be replaced once a year and the Exubera release units should be replaced every 2 weeks. The inhaler and blister doses should be stored at room temperature.
Dosage Forms: Exubera kit (should be used to initiate therapy): contains an inhaler, replacement chamber, 2 release units, 180 x 1-mg blisters, and 90 x 3-mg blisters. Exubera combination pack (should be used for subsequent refills): 90 x 1-mg blisters, 90 x 3-mg blisters, and 2 release units; or 180 x 1-mg blisters, 90 x 3-mg blisters, and 2 release units.
Website: www.exubera.com

Metformin (Glucophage/Glucophage XR, Glumetza, Fortamet)

Class: Biguanide
Mechanism of Action: Increases insulin sensitivity in the liver by inhibiting hepatic gluconeogenesis and/or glycogenolysis, thereby reducing hepatic glucose production. Metformin also enhances muscle glucose uptake and utilization.
Clinical Effects: Metformin reduces HbA1c by up to 1.5-2% and fasting blood glucose by up to 60-80 mg/dL.
Dosage: 500 mg tablet: starting dose is 500 mg twice a day with the morning and evening meals, up to a maximum of 2500 mg/day. 850 mg tablet: starting dose is 850 mg once daily with the largest meal, up to a maximum of 2550 mg/day. Dosage increases should be made in increments of one tablet every 2 weeks, up to a maximum of 2500 mg/day (2550 mg with 850 mg tablets).
Renal Impairment: Do not use in patients with renal insufficiency (serum creatinine ≥ 1.5 mg/dL in men or ≥ 1.4 mg/dL in women).
Hepatic Impairment: Do not use with severe liver disease.

Contraindications: Metformin should not be given to anyone ≥ 80 years of age without first documenting a normal creatinine clearance. Do not use in renal insufficiency (serum creatinine ≥ 1.5 mg/dL in men or ≥ 1.4 mg/dL in women), in patients receiving iodinated contrast material (discontinue temporarily for 48 hours after procedure because of potential for acute alteration of renal function, and do not resume until normal renal function has been documented), or in patients prone to metabolic acidosis or hypoxic states (liver failure, congestive heart failure requiring pharmacological therapy, diabetic ketoacidosis, major surgical procedures, sepsis, severe trauma, alcoholism, binge drinking, COPD); these conditions increase the risk of lactic acidosis.
Adverse Effects: Anorexia, nausea, abdominal discomfort, diarrhea, metallic taste, vitamin B_{12} deficiency, lactic acidosis.
Monitoring: Renal function, HbA1c, FBG, hematologic parameters (Hb, hematocrit, RBC indices).
Drug Interactions: Cimetidine increases blood levels of metformin.
Safety in Pregnancy: B
Comments: May be most useful in obese patients with dyslipidemia (decreases LDL and TG's); associated with no weight gain or mild weight loss. Approved for use down to 10 years of age.
Dosage Forms: Tablet: 500 mg, 850 mg, 1000 mg; Glucophage extended-release tablet: 500 mg, 750 mg; Glumetza extended-release tablet: 500 mg, 1000 mg
Website: www.pdr.net

Miglitol (Glyset)

Class: Alpha-glucosidase inhibitor
Mechanism of Action: These drugs act locally in the small intestine by inhibiting alpha-glucosidase enzymes; this action slows digestion of ingested carbohydrates, delays glucose absorption, and reduces the increase in postprandial blood glucose.
Dosage: 25 mg three times/day with the first bite of each main meal. Maintenance dose ranges are 50-100 mg three times/day. Dose adjustments should be made at 4-8 week intervals.
Clinical Effects: Alpha-glucosidase inhibitors cause a 0.5-1% reduction in HbA1c and have no significant effect on fasting blood glucose levels.
Renal Impairment: Primarily excreted by the kidneys; little information in patients with a CrCl < 25 mL/min.
Hepatic Impairment: No dosage adjustment is necessary.
Contraindications: Major GI disorders, including inflammatory bowel disease, chronic ulceration, malabsorption, or partial intestinal obstruction.
Adverse Effects: Abdominal bloating, flatulence, diarrhea, rash. Adverse GI effects tend to diminish with continued treatment.
Monitoring: HbA1c, FBG.
Drug Interactions: Decreases absorption and bioavailability of digoxin and propranolol; digestive enzymes (amylase, pancreatin),

intestinal adsorbents (charcoal) reduce effects of miglitol.
Safety in Pregnancy: B
Comments: Most effective in patients with postprandial hyperglycemia; not associated with weight gain or hypoglycemia; must use glucose and not complex sugars to reverse hypoglycemia, if it occurs
Dosage Forms: 25 mg, 50 mg, 100 mg tablets.
Website: www.glyset.com

Nateglinide (Starlix)

Class: Meglitinide (phenylalanine derivative)
Mechanism of Action: Meglitinides stimulate insulin release from pancreatic beta cells in response to a glucose load (meal). Insulin release is glucose dependent and diminishes at low glucose concentrations. There are distinct beta cell binding sites for nateglinide apart from the sulfonylurea binding site.
Clinical Effects: Nateglinide lowers HbA1c by up to 1% but has no significant effect on fasting blood glucose.
Dosage: Nateglinide has an initial and maintenance dose of 120 mg three times/day. If a patient is close to HbA1c goal, the dose may be started at 60 mg three times/day. Doses should be given 1-30 minutes before meals. The number of doses is based on the number of meals eaten. If a meal is skipped, that dose should be omitted. At least 1 week should elapse between dosage adjustments.
Renal Impairment: No dosage adjustment necessary.
Hepatic Impairment: Use with caution in patients with severe liver disease.
Contraindications: Hypersensitivity, type 1 diabetes, diabetic ketoacidosis with or without coma.
Adverse Effects: Hypoglycemia, headache, nausea, diarrhea, constipation, dizziness.
Monitoring: HbA1c, FBG.
Drug Interactions: No significant interactions.
Safety in Pregnancy: C
Comments: Most effective for lowering postprandial blood glucose.
Dosage Forms: 60 mg, 120 mg tablets.
Website: www.starlix.com

Pioglitazone (Actos)

Class: Thiazolidinedione
Mechanism of Action: Pioglitazone decreases insulin resistance in muscle and adipose tissue by activating the peroxisome proliferator-activated receptor gamma, which increases transcription of proteins involved in glucose uptake. It also decreases hepatic glucose production by improving hepatic insulin sensitivity, and preserves pancreatic beta-cell function.
Clinical Effects: Thiazolidinediones reduce HbA1c by up to 0.6-1.9 % and fasting blood glucose by up to 50-80 mg/dL.
Dosage: Pioglitazone has a starting dose of 15 mg/day with maintenance doses of 15-45 mg/day given as a single dose. May be given without regard to meals.

Renal Impairment: No dosage adjustment necessary.
Hepatic Impairment: Do not use in patients with active liver disease or increased serum transaminase levels (ALT > 2.5 x upper limit of normal).
Adverse Effects: Weight gain, edema, headache, myalgia, upper respiratory tract infection, anemia, macular edema (rare).
Warnings/Contraindications: Class III or IV heart failure (not recommended due to fluid retention), liver disease, type 1 diabetes (ineffective without insulin).
Drug Interactions: Effects of oral contraceptives and statins may be decreased based on data from another thiazolidinedione; additional caution regarding contraception is needed. Pioglitazone may be a weak inducer of CYP3A4.
Monitoring: HbA1c, FBG.
Safety in Pregnancy: C
Comments: May result in ovulation in premenopausal anovulatory women. It may take several weeks for onset of action and several months for peak activity. Requires the presence of insulin for action.
Dosage Forms: 15 mg, 30 mg, 45 mg tablets.
Website: www.actos.com

Pioglitazone/Glimepiride (Duetact)

Class: Thiazolidinedione/sulfonylurea
Mechanism of Action: Pioglitazone decreases insulin resistance in muscle and adipose tissue by activating the peroxisome proliferator-activated receptor gamma, which increases transcription of proteins involved in glucose uptake. It also decreases hepatic glucose production by improving hepatic insulin sensitivity. Sulfonylureas stimulate insulin secretion by blocking the potassium channel of the beta cell. They also decrease hepatic glucose production and may improve insulin sensitivity at the receptor and post-receptor levels.
Clinical Effects: When pioglitazone is added to a sulfonylurea, the fasting blood glucose is decreased by up to 40-60 mg/dL and the HbA1c is reduced by up to 0.9-1.7%.
Dosage: Initial dose is 30/2 mg once daily in patients previously on monotherapy with a sulfonylurea or pioglitazone. May increase dose at 1-2 week intervals, but in patients previously treated with sulfonylurea monotherapy, it may take 2-3 months to see the full effect of the pioglitazone component. Maximum recommended daily dose is 45 mg of pioglitazone and 8 mg of glimepiride.
Renal Impairment: Initial dosing should be conservative.
Hepatic Impairment: Do not use in patients with active liver disease or increased serum transaminase levels (ALT > 2.5 x upper limit of normal).
Warnings and Contraindications: Class III or IV heart failure (not recommended due to fluid retention), liver disease, type 1 diabetes mellitus (ineffective without insulin), diabetic ketoacidosis.
Adverse Effects: Weight gain, edema, fluid retention, hypoglycemia, headache,

dizziness, weakness, nausea, myalgia, macular edema (rare).

Drug Interactions: Effects of oral contraceptives and statins may be decreased; additional caution regarding contraception is needed. Pioglitazone may be a weak inducer of CYP3A4.

Monitoring: HbA1c, FBG.

Safety in Pregnancy: C

Comments: May result in ovulation in premenopausal anovulatory women. It may take several weeks for onset of action and several months for peak activity of pioglitazone component. Should be given once daily with the first meal of the day.

Dosage Forms: 30/2 mg, 30/4 mg tablets

Website: www.duetact.com

Pioglitazone/Metformin (ACTOplusMet)

Class: Thiazolidinedione/biguanide

Mechanism of Action: Pioglitazone decreases insulin resistance in muscle and adipose tissue by activating the peroxisome proliferator-activated receptor gamma, which increases transcription of proteins involved in glucose uptake. It also decreases hepatic glucose production by improving hepatic insulin sensitivity. Metformin increases insulin sensitivity in the liver by inhibiting hepatic gluconeogenesis and/or glycogenolysis, thereby reducing hepatic glucose production. It also enhances muscle glucose uptake and utilization.

Clinical Effects: When pioglitazone is added to metformin, the fasting blood glucose is decreased by up to 40-50 mg/dL and the HbA1c is reduced by up to 1%.

Dosage: Initial dose is 15/500 mg or 15/850 mg once or twice daily with meals in patients on metformin monotherapy. For patients on pioglitazone monotherapy, the initial dose should be 15/500 mg twice daily or 15/850 mg once daily. Patients switching from combination therapy with pioglitazone plus metformin as separate tablets may be started on either the 15/500 mg or 15/850 mg tablet strengths based on the doses of each medication already being taken. Doses should be given with meals and titrated gradually. Maximum recommended daily dose is 45 mg of pioglitazone and 2550 mg of metformin.

Renal Impairment: Do not use in patients with renal insufficiency (serum creatinine ≥ 1.5 mg/dL in men or ≥ 1.4 mg/dL in women).

Hepatic Impairment: Do not use in patients with active liver disease or increased serum transaminase levels (ALT > 2.5 x upper limit of normal).

Contraindications: Metformin should not be given to anyone ≥ 80 years of age without first documenting a normal creatinine clearance. Because of the metformin component, do not use in renal insufficiency (serum creatinine ≥ 1.5 mg/dL in men or ≥ 1.4 mg/dL in women); in patients receiving iodinated contrast material (discontinue temporarily for 48 hours after procedure because of potential for acute alteration of renal function, and do not resume until normal renal function has been documented); or in patients prone to metabolic acidosis or hypoxic states (liver failure, congestive heart failure requiring pharmacological therapy, diabetic ketoacidosis, major surgical procedures, sepsis, severe trauma, alcoholism, binge drinking, COPD); these conditions increase the risk of developing lactic acidosis. Not recommended for type 1 diabetes, Class III or IV heart failure (due to fluid retention).

Adverse Effects: Weight gain, edema, fluid retention, myalgia, nausea, anorexia, abdominal discomfort, diarrhea, metallic taste, vitamin B12 deficiency, lactic acidosis, macular edema (rare).

Drug Interactions: Effects of oral contraceptives and statins may be decreased by pioglitazone; additional caution regarding contraception is needed. Pioglitazone may also be a weak inducer of CYP3A4. Cimetidine increases blood levels of metformin.

Monitoring: HbA1c, FBG, renal function, hematologic parameters (Hb, hematocrit, RBC indices).

Safety in Pregnancy: C

Comments: May result in ovulation in premenopausal anovulatory women. It may take several weeks for onset of action and several months for peak activity of pioglitazone component.

Dosage Forms: 15/500 mg, 15/850 mg tablets

Website: www.actoplusmet.com

Pramlintide (Symlin)

Class: Amylin mimetic

Mechanism of Action: Amylin is a neuroendocrine hormone secreted with insulin by pancreatic beta cells in response to food intake and subsequent elevations in blood glucose. Pramlintide is an amylin mimetic that slows gastric emptying, reducing the rate at which glucose appears in the bloodstream; decreases postprandial hepatic glucose output by suppressing glucagon secretion; and decreases food intake by enhancing satiety, potentially leading to weight loss.

Clinical Effects: Type 1 diabetes: Lowers HbA1c by 0.18-0.33%, reduces weight by 1.1-3.0 kg, and reduces total, short-acting, and long-acting insulin by up to 12%, 21.7%, and 0.4%, respectively. Type 2 diabetes: Lowers HbA1c by 0.4-0.56%, reduces weight by 1.5-2.76 kg, reduces total, short-acting, and long-acting insulin by up to 6.4%, 10.3%, and 4.2%, respectively.

Dosage: Type 1 diabetes: Starting dose is 15 mcg subcutaneously before each major meal (at least 250 calories or 30 gm carbohydrates). Reduce pre-meal insulin dose (rapid-acting, short-acting, and fixed-mix [70/30] insulin) by 50%. Increase pramlintide in 15 mcg increments to a maintenance dose of 30-60 mcg before major meals. Dose increases should be made when there is no nausea for 3 days. If nausea persists at the 45 or 60 mcg doses, reduce dose to 30 mcg. If the 30 mcg dose is not tolerated, consider discontinuing. Adjust insulin dose once patient is on a stable pramlintide regimen.

Type 2 diabetes: Starting dose is 60 mcg subcutaneously before each major meal (at least 250 calories or 30 gm carbohydrates). Reduce pre-meal insulin dose (rapid-acting, short-acting, and fixed-mix [70/30] insulin) by 50%.

Increase pramlintide to 120 mcg when there is no nausea for 3-7 days. If nausea persists at the 120 mcg dose, reduce dose to 60 mcg. Adjust insulin dose once patient is on a stable pramlintide regimen.

Administration: Pramlintide and insulin should always be administered as separate injections. It should not be mixed with any type of insulin and should be given subcutaneously into the abdomen or thigh.

Renal Impairment: No dosage adjustment is necessary if creatinine clearance >20 mL/min. Has not been studied in patients on hemodialysis.

Hepatic Impairment: Not studied in patients with hepatic insufficiency. Hepatic dysfunction is not expected to affect blood concentrations since pramlintide undergoes mostly renal metabolism.

Monitoring: HbA1c, FBG.

Warnings/Contraindications: Pramlintide is used with insulin and has been associated with an increased risk of insulin-induced hypoglycemia, particularly in patients with Type 1 diabetes. When severe hypoglycemia with pramlintide occurs, it is seen within 3 hours following a pramlintide injection. Appropriate patient selection, careful patient instruction, and insulin dose adjustments are critical elements for reducing this risk. Contraindications include hypersensitivity to pramlintide or any of its components, including metacresol; gastroparesis; hypoglycemia unawareness.

Adverse Effects: Hypoglycemia, nausea, headache, anorexia, vomiting, abdominal pain, fatigue

Drug Interactions: Due to its effects on gastric emptying, pramlintide should not be used with drugs that alter gastrointestinal motility or slow intestinal absorption. It may delay the absorption of oral medications taken concurrently, so if a drug requires a rapid onset or is dependent on threshold concentrations for efficacy, such as levothyroxine, it should be taken 1 hour prior to or 2 hours after pramlintide is given.

Safety in Pregnancy: C

Comments: Pramlintide is indicated as an adjunct treatment for type 1 diabetes patients who use mealtime insulin and have failed to achieve adequate glycemic control. It is also indicated for type 2 diabetes patients who use mealtime insulin and have failed to achieve adequate glycemic control, with or without a concurrent sulfonylurea and/or metformin.

Dosage Forms: 5 ml vial (60 mcg/mL). Unopened vials should be kept refrigerated prior to use. The vial may be kept at room temperature or refrigerated once opened and should be used within 28 days.

Website: www.symlin.com

Repaglinide (Prandin)

Class: Meglitinide (benzoic acid derivative)

Mechanism of Action: Meglitinides stimulate insulin release from pancreatic beta cells in response to a glucose load (meal). Insulin release is glucose dependent and diminishes at low glucose concentrations. There are distinct beta cell binding sites for repaglinide apart from the sulfonylurea binding site.

Clinical Effects: Repaglinidc lowers HbA1c by up to 1-2% and fasting blood glucose by up to 60-80 mg/dL.

Dosage: For patients not previously treated or whose HbA1c < 8%, the starting dose should be 0.5 mg with each meal; if patient has previously been treated with blood-glucose lowering agents or whose HbA1c > 8%, the initial dose is 1 or 2 mg with each meal. The dosage range is 0.5-4 mg with each meal (maximum daily dose = 16 mg). The number of doses is based on the number of meals eaten, and should be given within 15 minutes of each meal. If a meal is skipped, that dose should be omitted. At least 1 week should elapse between dosage adjustments.

Renal Impairment: CrCl = 20-40 mL/min: initiate with 0.5 mg with meals and titrate carefully.

Hepatic Impairment: Use conservative initial and maintenance doses; use longer intervals between dose adjustments.

Contraindications: Hypersensitivity, type 1 diabetes, diabetic ketoacidosis with or without coma.

Adverse Effects: Hypoglycemia, headache, nausea/vomiting/diarrhea, constipation, dyspepsia.

Monitoring: HbA1c, FBG.

Drug Interactions: CYP2C9 and CYP3A3/4 enzyme substrate. Agents that inhibit or induce these enzymes may increase repaglinide concentrations. Gemfibrozil and itraconazole increase levels of repaglinide (not recommended for concurrent use).

Safety in Pregnancy: C

Comments: Most effective for decreasing postprandial blood glucose

Dosage Forms: 0.5 mg, 1 mg, 2 mg tablets.

Website: www.prandin.com

Rosiglitazone (Avandia)

Class: Thiazolidinedione

Mechanism of Action: Rosiglitazone decreases insulin resistance in muscle and adipose tissue by activating the peroxisome proliferator-activated receptor gamma, which increases transcription of proteins involved in glucose uptake. It also decreases hepatic glucose production by improving hepatic insulin sensitivity, and preserves pancreatic beta-cell function.

Clinical Effects: Thiazolidinediones reduce HbA1c by up to 0.6-1.9 % and fasting blood glucose by up to 50-80 mg/dL.

Dosage: Rosiglitazone has a starting dose of 4 mg/day, with maintenance doses of 2-8 mg/day given in 1 or 2 divided doses. Dosage increases may be made if patients have inadequate response following 8-12 weeks of treatment.

Renal Impairment: No dose adjustment necessary.

Hepatic Impairment: Do not use if patient has active live disease or

increased serum transaminase levels (ALT > 2.5 x upper limit of normal).
Monitoring: HbA1c, FBG.
Drug Interactions: Gemfibrozil and other inhibitors of CYP2C8 may increase rosiglitazone concentrations; rifampin and other inducers of CYP2C8 may decrease rosiglitazone concentrations.
Warnings/Contraindications: Class III or IV heart failure (not recommended due to fluid retention), liver disease, type 1 diabetes mellitus (ineffective without insulin).
Adverse Effects: Weight gain, fluid retention, headache, anemia, macular edema (rare).
Safety in Pregnancy: C
Comments: It may take several weeks for onset of action and several months for peak activity. Requires the presence of insulin for action. Approved for use in triple combination therapy (with secretagogue plus metformin).
Dosage Forms: 2 mg, 4 mg, 8 mg tablets.
Website: www.avandia.com

Rosiglitazone/Glimepiride (Avandaryl)

Class: Thiazolidinedione/sulfonylurea
Mechanism of Action: Rosiglitazone decreases insulin resistance in muscle and adipose tissue by activating the peroxisome proliferator-activated receptor gamma, which increases transcription of proteins involved in glucose uptake. It also decreases hepatic glucose production by improving hepatic insulin sensitivity. Sulfonylureas stimulate insulin secretion by blocking the potassium channel of the beta cell. They also decrease hepatic glucose production and may improve insulin sensitivity at the receptor and post-receptor levels.
Clinical Effects: When rosiglitazone is added to a sulfonylurea, the fasting blood glucose is decreased by up to 40-65 mg/dL and the HbA1c is reduced by up to 0.9-1.5%.
Dosage: Initial dose is 4/1 mg or 4/2 mg once daily in patients previously on monotherapy with a sulfonylurea or rosiglitazone. For patients previously treated with rosiglitazone monotherapy, the dose of Avandaryl may be increased by increasing the glimepiride component in no more than 2 mg increments at 1-2 week intervals. For patients previously treated with sulfonylurea monotherapy, it may take 2 weeks to see a reduction in blood glucose and 2-3 months to see the full effect of the rosiglitazone component. If additional glucose control is needed, the dose of the glimepiride component may be increased. Maximum recommended daily dose is 8 mg of rosiglitazone and 4 mg of glimepiride.
Renal Impairment: Initial dosing should be conservative.
Hepatic Impairment: Do not use in patients with active liver disease or increased serum transaminases (ALT > 2.5 x upper limit of normal).
Warnings and Contraindications: Class III or IV heart failure (not recommended due to fluid retention), liver disease, type 1 diabetes mellitus

(ineffective without insulin), diabetic ketoacidosis.
Adverse Effects: Weight gain, fluid retention, hypoglycemia, headache, dizziness, weakness, nausea, macular edema (rare).
Drug Interactions: Gemfibrozil increases rosiglitazone concentrations; rifampin decreases rosiglitazone concentrations.
Monitoring: HbA1c, FBG.
Safety in Pregnancy: C
Comments: May result in ovulation in premenopausal anovulatory women. It may take several weeks for onset of action and several months for peak activity of rosiglitazone component.
Dosage Forms: 4/1 mg, 4/2 mg, 4/4 mg tablets
Website: www.avandaryl.com

Rosiglitazone/Metformin (Avandamet)

Class: Thiazolidinedione/biguanide
Mechanism of Action: Rosiglitazone decreases insulin resistance in muscle and adipose tissue by activating the peroxisome proliferator-activated receptor-gamma, which increases transcription of proteins involved in glucose uptake. It also decreases hepatic glucose production by improving hepatic insulin sensitivity, and preserves pancreatic beta-cell function.
Metformin increases insulin sensitivity in the liver by inhibiting hepatic gluconeogenesis and/or glycogenolysis, thereby reducing hepatic glucose production. It also enhances muscle glucose uptake and utilization.
Dosage: If patient's metformin dose was 1000 mg/day, start with 2/500 mg twice a day with meals. If patient's metformin dose was 2000 mg/day, start with 2/1000 mg twice a day with meals. If patient's rosiglitazone dose was 4 mg/day, start with 2/500 mg twice a day with meals. If patient's rosiglitazone dose was 8 mg/day, start with 4/500 mg twice a day with meals. If patients have inadequate response, metformin dosage increases may be made after 1-2 weeks and rosiglitazone dosage increases may be made after 8-12 weeks of treatment. Maximum recommended daily dose is 8/2000 mg.
Renal Impairment: Metformin should not be given to anyone over the age of 80 without first documenting a normal creatinine clearance. Because of the metformin component, do not use in patients with renal insufficiency (serum creatinine ≥ 1.5 mg/dL in men or ≥ 1.4 mg/dL in women).
Hepatic Impairment: Do not use if patient has active live disease or increased serum transaminase levels (ALT > 2.5x upper limit of normal).
Monitoring: HbA_{1c}, FBG, renal function, hematologic parameters.
Drug Interactions: Gemfibrozil increases rosiglitazone concentrations; rifampin decreases rosiglitazone concentrations.
Warnings and Contraindications: Class III or IV heart failure (not recommended due to fluid retention), liver disease, type 1 diabetes mellitus (ineffective without insulin), acute or chronic metabolic acidosis. Others include renal insufficiency (serum

creatinine ≥ 1.5 mg/dL in men or ≥ 1.4 mg/dL in women), patients receiving iodinated contrast material (discontinue temporarily for 48 hours after procedure because of potential for acute alteration of renal function, and do not resume until normal renal function has been documented), patients prone to metabolic acidosis or hypoxic states (liver failure, congestive heart failure requiring pharmacological therapy, diabetic ketoacidosis, major surgical procedures, sepsis, severe trauma, alcoholism, binge drinking, COPD); these conditions increase the risk of lactic acidosis.

Adverse Effects: Weight gain, fluid retention, hepatotoxicity, anemia, headache, anorexia, nausea, abdominal discomfort, diarrhea, metallic taste, vitamin B_{12} deficiency, lactic acidosis, macular edema (rare).

Safety in Pregnancy: C

Comments: May result in ovulation in premenopausal anovulatory women. It may take several weeks for onset of action and several months for peak activity. Requires the presence of insulin for action.

Dosage Forms: 1/500 mg, 2/500 mg, 4/500 mg, 2/1000 mg, 4/1000 mg tablets.

Website: www.avandamet.com

Sitagliptin (Januvia)

Class: Dipeptidyl peptidase-4 (DPP-4) inhibitor

Mechanism of Action: Glucagon-like peptide-1 (GLP-1) and glucose-dependent insulinotropic polypeptide (GIP) are incretin hormones that are released from cells in the intestine in response to food. They bind to receptors on pancreatic beta cells, stimulating the release of insulin and reducing the release of glucagon. Sitagliptin works by inhibiting DPP-4, an enzyme that rapidly breaks down GLP-1 and GIP. The incretin system is impaired in type 2 diabetics, so sitagliptin enhances its function, leading to decreased blood sugar levels as well as preserving beta-cell function.

Clinical Efficacy: Sitagliptin reduces HbA_{1c} by 0.7-1.5% when used as monotherapy and by up to 2.9% when used in combination with metformin or a thiazolidinedione. It also decreases fasting blood glucose by up to 25 mg/dL.

Dosage: 100 mg once daily as monotherapy or in combination with metformin or a thiazolidinedione.

Renal Impairment: CrCl 30-50 mL/min: 50 mg/day; CrCl < 30 mL/min or ESRD (on dialysis): 25 mg/day.

Hepatic Impairment: No dosage adjustment necessary.

Adverse Effects: Nasopharyngitis, headache, upper respiratory tract infection.

Monitoring: HbA_{1c}, FBG, renal function.

Drug Interactions: Slight increase in digoxin concentrations in patients on 100 mg dose of sitagliptin.

Safety in Pregnancy: B

Comments: Not associated with weight gain.

Dosage Forms: 25 mg, 50 mg, 100 mg tablets.

Website: www.januvia.com

Vildagliptin (Galvus)

Class: Dipeptidyl peptidase-IV (DPP-4) inhibitor
Mechanism of Action: Glucagon-like peptide-1 (GLP-1) and glucose-dependent insulinotropic polypeptide (GIP) are incretin hormones that are released from cells in the intestine in response to food. They bind to receptors on pancreatic beta cells, stimulating the release of insulin and reducing the release of glucagon. Vildagliptin works by inhibiting DPP-4, an enzyme that rapidly breaks down GLP-1 and GIP. The incretin system is impaired in type 2 diabetics, so vildagliptin enhances its function, leading to decreased blood sugar levels as well as preserving beta-cell function.
Clinical Efficacy: Vildagliptin reduces HbA_{1c} by 0.7-1.9% when used as monotherapy and by up to 2.8% when used in combination with metformin or a thiazolidinedione. It also decreases fasting blood glucose by up to 25 mg/dL.
Dosage: Expected dose is 100 mg daily as monotherapy or in combination with metformin or a thiazolidinedione.
Renal Impairment: Not available at press time, but dose reductions in patients with renal insufficiency are expected.
Hepatic Impairment: No dosage adjustment necessary.
Adverse Effects: Nasopharyngitis, headache, upper respiratory tract infection.
Monitoring: HbA_{1c}, FBG, renal function.
Drug Interactions: None known.
Safety in Pregnancy: B
Comments: Not associated with weight gain.
Website: www.galvus.com

Insulin*

Mechanism of Action: Main hormone required for proper glucose utilization and metabolic processes. Categorized by onset, duration, and intensity of action
Adverse Effects: Hypoglycemia, local reactions (itching, edema, stinging, pain or warmth at injection site, atrophy or hypertrophy of subcutaneous fat tissue).
Safety in Pregnancy: B, except for glargine (Lantus), detemir (Levemir), aspart (Novolog) and glulisine (Apidra), which are category C.
Compatibility of Insulin Preparations, Timing of Administration, Dosage Forms (Injections): See Tables 11.1 and 11.2, pp. 173-174.
Website: www.pdr.net

* Also see p. 160 for inhaled human insulin (Exubera)

Table 11.1. Insulin Products

Insulin	Onset	Peak	Duration
Rapid-acting			
Lispro (Humulog)	5-15 min	30-90 min	5 h
Aspart (Novolog)	5-15 min	30-90 min	5 h
Glulisine (Apidra)	5-15 min	30-90 min	5 h
Inhaled (Exubera)	10-20 min	30-90 min	5-8 h
Short-acting			
Regular U100 (Humulin R/Novolin R)	30-60 min	2-3 h	5-8 h
Regular U500 (concentrated)	30-60 min	2-3 h	5-8 h
Intermediate-acting			
Isophane insulin (NPH = Humulin N/Novolin N)	2-4 h	4-10 h	10-16 h
Long-acting			
Glargine (Lantus)	2-4 h	no peak	20-24 h
Detemir (Levemir)	2-4 h	6-8 h	6-23 h
Premixed			
70% NPH/30% regular (Humulin 70/30, Novolin 70/30)	30-60 min	dual	10-16 h
50% NPH/50% regular (Humulin 50/50)	30-60 min	dual	10-16 h
75% NPL/25% lispro (Humulog Mix 75/25)	5-15 min	dual	10-16 h
50% NPL/50% lispro (Humulog Mix 50/50)	5-15 min	dual	10-16 h
70% NPA/30% aspart (Novolog Mix)	5-15 min	dual	10-16 h

NPH = neutral protamine Hagedorn, NPL = insulin lispro protamine, NPA = insulin aspart protamine. Adapted from: JAMA 2003;289:2254-2264.

Table 11.2. Compatibility and Timing of Insulin Products

Compatibility of Insulin Preparations
Lispro (Humulog): Compatible with NPH
Aspart (Novolog): Compatible with NPH
Regular insulin: Compatible with NPH if given ≤ 5 minutes after mixing
Isophane insulin suspension (NPH): Compatible with regular insulin, lispro, aspart
Glargine (Lantus): Should not be mixed with other insulins
Timing of Administration
Rapid-acting (lispro, aspart, glulisine, inhaled): Given 1-15 min before a meal (usually 5 min)
Short-acting (regular): Given 30-60 min before a meal
Intermediate-acting (NPH): Given 2 times per day
Long-acting (glargine, detemir): Given once a day

Table 11.3. Approximate Guidelines for Initial Pre-meal Exubera Dose*

Patient Weight (kg)	Patient Weight (lb)	Initial Dose per Meal	Number of 1-mg blisters per dose	Number of 3-mg blisters per dose
30 - 39.9	66 - 87	1 mg	1	–
40 - 59.9	88 - 132	2 mg	2	–
60 - 79.9	133 - 176	3 mg	–	1
80 - 99.9	177 - 220	4 mg	1	1
100 - 119.9	221 - 264	5 mg	2	1
120 - 139.9	265 - 308	6 mg	–	2

* See p. 160 for Exubera drug summary.

From: U.S. Package Insert. www.exubera.com.

Index

DIABETES ESSENTIALS — ORDERING INFORMATION

Price (U.S. dollars)

1–9 copies:	$17.95 each
10–49 copies:	$16.95 each
50–100 copies:	$15.95 each
> 100 copies:	call

Shipping

USA: UPS Ground delivery (call for next day, 2-day, or 3-day express delivery charges):

1–3 copies:	add $5
4–10 copies:	add $7
10–49 copies:	add $12
> 50 copies:	call

Outside USA: Call, fax, or e-mail for delivery charges

Michigan residents: add 6%

4 Ways to Order:

By Phone:	(248) 616-3023
By Fax:*	(248) 616-3003
By Mail:*	Physicians' Press 620 Cherry Avenue Royal Oak, Michigan 48073
By Internet:	www.physicianspress.com

* Please print or type name, mailing address, credit card number and expiration date or purchase order number (if applicable), telephone number (important), fax number, and e-mail address. We accept VISA, MasterCard, and American Express.